Living with the Bully of Crohn's Disease

James Patterson

Copyright © 2014 James Patterson

All rights reserved.

ISBN: 1495415759
ISBN-13: 978-1495415753

DISCLAIMER

The opinions expressed in this book are my own and based upon my own ideas and personal experiences as a Crohn's patient for over 47 years. This is what I have lived through. The information presented here are my attempts to improve my health and manage a difficult and unrelenting medical disease that has significantly affected my life. It may not apply to the reader and is not a substitute for your doctor's medical care or advice. I am not licensed to practice medicine; I do not have a medical degree; I am not licensed or trained in psychology or psychiatry; and I am not a member of the clergy or affiliated with any religious or spiritual institution. Do not disregard medical advice or delay seeking medical care based upon anything you may read in this book.

CONTENTS

    Acknowledgements

1. My Story —Year of Sickness without a Diagnosis — 1
2. Gathering My Healthcare Team — 13
3. Finding Personal Support — 22
4. Managing Crohn's —Pills, Potions, Diet and More — 31
5. When Surgery becomes Necessary — 47
6. Psychological Help — 63
7. Using the Mind for First Aid — 69
8. The Bully of Crohn's Disease — 86
9. Relief from Intimidating Fear — 96
10. Cooling Inflammatory Anger — 108
11. Managing Immobilizing Guilt — 115
12. Dealing with Distorted Beliefs — 125
13. Therapeutic Gratitude — 145
14. Healing with Forgiveness — 154
15. Creating Joy — 170
16. Spiritual Help — 180
17. The Search for New and Better Answers — 195

ACKNOWLEDGMENTS

I want to express my heartfelt gratitude to my wife Mary Lou for her many years of support and help in dealing with the Bully of Crohn's disease. She has been by my side through all of it, spent many a night in the ER or the hospital, listened to my complaints and tales of woe, comforted me when I was at my wit's end and through it all, she has supplied me with her kindness, insights, and love.

I am grateful to my family and friends who have sent me their best wishes and prayers over the years along with words of encouragement and support.

I have many health care professionals; they all have been great listeners and have done their best to help me through difficult times. They were my champions as they worked with me on new ideas to manage my physical pain and difficulties. They were patient as they spent many hours trying to improve my quality of life.

Finally, I wish to give special thanks to one particular physician friend who was instrumental in my initial diagnosis of Crohn's disease and talked with me about the mental and emotional components of disease processes. He opened my eyes to the idea that there is more to health than just a healthy body. My health includes emotional, mental, and spiritual components and these have a profound impact on both my physical health and my overall sense of well-being and peace. His insights were instrumental in sending me down the path of improved health and served as the motivation behind many of the ideas in this book.

Chapter 1— My Story —Years of Sickness without a Diagnosis

My first symptoms of Crohn's disease appeared when I was thirteen years old. My diagnosis came 38 years later. To put that span of time in perspective, my family bought our first color television set when I was thirteen. By the time of my diagnosis, I could watch color TV and make a phone call on a device that fit into my shirt pocket.

My "stomach" area has been sensitive for as long as I can remember. Eating food and digesting it easily was a problem since my grammar school days. In my case, the initial significant manifestations of Crohn's disease were bleeding and pain. As a teenager, the discovery of the bleeding and pain secured a referral to a proctologist and he found ulcerations. Looking back, these ulcerations were early Crohn's disease but nobody knew this at that time. The treatment was a chemical burn or cauterization with silver nitrate. After six to seven treatments, the bleeding stopped and I was considered "healed."

My family spent a lot of time vacationing at the beach in Baja, California, where I was ill on a regular basis. Nobody else in the family had issues or illness but they assumed I had ingested contaminated food or water. A local physician treated me for food or water poisoning but it never helped my symptoms and nobody suspected Crohn's disease.

Time passed. I married a wonderful woman; we had two beautiful daughters. I finished graduate school and started a highly successful career in medical diagnostics. I was busy with work, outdoor activities, and family time. However, I noticed new symptoms including a fiery type of abdominal pain, fever, abdominal cramps, and spasms. My wardrobe changed because tight-waisted pants became too painful to wear as they rubbed on my stomach. Sleeping on my stomach was out of the question, and my energy sagged. My repeated visits to the doctor resulted in stress-related diagnoses. They recommended antidepressants, counseling, meditation, and relaxation as possible therapies for my stress and I tried them all with limited results. I learned to adjust my daily schedule to accommodate the pain and lack of energy with my feverish symptoms. I curtailed my bike riding, surfing, racquetball, and other heavy physical activities that I had previously enjoyed.

At one point, I had a revealing experience as I underwent a small surgery to repair a chronic bleeding fissure. I was given a spinal block and remained awake through the procedure. I can still recall the blessed relief of not being able to feel anything below my waist. With each deep inhalation, my lungs would expand and then contract and there was no pain. I reveled in this feeling and took deep, relaxed breaths throughout the procedure. The back of my head, my upper back, and my eyes also felt comfortable and relaxed. It became obvious to me that the constant gastrointestinal (GI) pain that had accompanied me for years was not only creating pain in my gut but was creating pain and discomfort in other parts of my body. In response to this pain, my body was in a constant state of tension. This vivid memory has remained with me for decades and is a constant reminder that the gut pain associated with Crohn's disease influences my sense of comfort far beyond my GI system.

In later years, a routine visit to my physician revealed that I was anemic—specifically, iron deficiency anemia—and I woke up one morning with a new pain in my gut. This intense mid-epigastric pain bored right through to my back and made it impossible to stand up. My trip to the emergency room resulted in a diagnosis of acute pancreatitis. This was unusual because I do not drink. The ER staff put me through my first of many CT scans and the only image of note was some unusual-looking bowel loops. This was attributed to normal peristalsis (wavelike movement of the intestines) and dismissed as clinically insignificant. Years later, it was obvious this was stricturing (severe narrowing of the intestines) and Crohn's disease was the culprit.

My saga continued with more bouts of pancreatitis, elevated liver enzymes, weight loss, pain and anemia. I learned to sleep while sitting in a lounge chair because I could not lie down without pain. Each morning brought uncertainty and fear as I wondered if I would get through the day or end up in the Emergency room, vomiting, or in the bathroom doubled up in agony. There were times away from home when my pain became extreme and I had to find a place to lie down in bathrooms, in the park, in hallways, or in my car and hope the pain would subside. My diet was rice crackers and blenderized low fiber foods because that was all I could tolerate. Social trips in the evening were always done on an empty stomach. If we were going out, I would stop eating 4-5 hours before the event. There was no eating on an airplane, while taking a long car trip, with our friends or family, or going off to the beach for the day. I ate enough to survive; anything more than that carried the risk of more pain, obstructions, or a run to the bathroom.

Finally, 32 years after my initial symptoms, my doctor gave me my first referral to see a gastroenterologist. An endoscopy revealed severe inflammation and ulcerations in the duodenum and proximal jejunum. The diagnosis was celiac disease (which is intolerance to gluten that is found in wheat, rye, and barley) and I was placed on a gluten-free diet (which I remain on to this day.) In a concerted effort to address my eight upper GI strictures, I received endoscopies with balloon dilations on a regular basis that went on for years. One of the dilations resulted in a perforated bowel and required a major emergency surgery.

In June of 2004, I continued to suffer from regular bleeding and anemia. My gluten-free diet was unsuccessful in curing my symptoms. Every day I used heating pads and took hot baths in an attempt to manage the constant abdominal pain. I would sit in a chair for hours because I felt so ill. I slept poorly and felt anxious and depressed. I came to fear the thought, "Would I be able to carry with any semblance of a normal life?" I worried about holding my job, taking care of my family, and being a good spouse, father, or friend. Nausea was a constant in my life and food and celebrations involving food flooded me with despair, sadness, and anxiety. I even wondered if I would be alive in the near future as I constantly struggled to maintain my weight and each day seemed to bring a new disappointment or pain. The mental consternation associated with decades of no answers was depressing.

Around this time, I spoke to a physician friend about my challenges. He thought about it for a moment and suggested this was not Celiac disease but something else. With this new thought, I contacted the pathologists who had previously read my tissue biopsy "glass slides." I was fortunate enough to find and collect about 20 of these slides that another pathologist could re-read. I located a group of specialized GI pathologists at a major medical center in Los Angeles who agreed to view these pathology slides. I delivered the slides to their practice and several days later they sent a report that stated I did not have Celiac disease. Their best interpretation of my ailment was Crohn's disease.

Armed with this new finding, I called an acquaintance who worked for a commercial company that focused on IBD and Crohn's disease. He gave me the name of the best Crohn's doctor in the area and then personally called to secure me an appointment. This doctor later examined me and verified I had Crohn's disease. With an independent diagnosis by a clinician and pathologist who specialized in Crohn's disease, my ailment was finally identified. My trail of previous diagnoses included stress-related anxiety, hypochondria, depression, bleeding ulcers (of unknown etiology), irritable bowel syndrome, fever syndrome (of unknown etiology), iron-deficient anemia (of unknown etiology), pancreatitis (of unknown etiology), elevated liver enzymes (of, you guessed it, unknown etiology), Celiac disease, and finally Crohn's disease.

I would like to admit my diagnosis 38 years later resulted in some exceptional treatments and control of the disease. However, the path to healing even after the diagnosis was a slow one.

The next seven years were my attempt to find a treatment plan that worked. There were more procedures, surgeries, hospitalizations, IV feedings, iron infusions, liquid diets, and ER visits. My doctors knew what we were dealing with but were unable to bring it under control due to the significant damage done to my bowels and the refractory nature of my ailment.

The balance of this book is my attempt to communicate what I learned about managing Crohn's disease, the many tools I created, and how others helped me. While it has been a difficult journey, I am fortunate to have many good people in my life who helped temper my distress. My disease is still present, but it is under better control due to the efforts of many. I have learned that my life can be healthier and more fruitful—but I must keep a constant surveillance on Crohn's and work with many tools to handle the physical and psychological damage. Crohn's is not something I can ignore and just hope it goes away.

Reflecting on my 38-year journey to diagnosis, I have tried to recognize what I gained from those nearly four decades of hard-fought wisdom in looking for a diagnosis. I knew there must be ideas and learning experiences that I could commit to memory for possible use in the future for others or myself. While Crohn's disease can be difficult to diagnose, earlier diagnosis is critical to achieve the best results. Below are some of the lessons I learned from my delayed diagnosis.

1. *I made a mistake in not taking my symptoms more seriously. I took them too lightly or too readily accepted them.*

I should have aggressively pursued answers in the face of my dismal improvement. My search for solutions was too passive. By tolerating my condition and not being more persistent, I prolonged my misdiagnosis. I am the most knowledgeable person when it comes to my own mind and body and it is important for me to observe how differently I feel from day to day or month to month. By noting these differences, I can use them to pursue new actions and take better care of myself.

I should have used my common sense as I asked myself the following questions: Did I see others sleeping in a chair because it was too painful to lie down? Did other people have unusual bowel movements? Did other people use Tylenol or heavier drugs as a part of their daily routine for GI pain? Did other people have serious pain or vomit after eating a meal? The answer is no, these are not common experiences in normal people.

I could have approached my symptoms and observed how often they occurred. If they happened occasionally, this might be normal or a response to a passing situation. I could have observed if my pain was a new symptom or if I noticed it before, if it was growing in intensity or fading away. However, since my symptoms were occurring all the time that should have been my warning signs that this was something more serious. I could have used this information and followed up with my physician. This lesson has taught me that my health is not up to my doctor, family, employer, or friend. I need to take charge of my own health.

2. *Not doing anything about a physical ailment is a bad option.*

This resulted in a much more serious medical condition. My decades of non-treatment resulted in a significant amount of tissue damage, which in turn has required more invasive and traumatic treatment options. In addition, it drastically affected my life for years as I missed many family activities and times of celebration. I also suffered more than was necessary—including significant mental suffering caused by my self-doubt, frustration, and fear. An earlier diagnosis would have saved me from agonizing about what was wrong and why I experienced chronic physical pain. Much of my own nervousness and mental confusion was due to my unrelenting discomfort from this ailment.

3. *I let too much time pass between follow-up visits with my clinician.*

I did not see my doctor after a reasonable time when there was no improvement. I had bought into the idea that both the origins and manifestations of my symptoms were strictly psychological with no physiological and biological root. My good friends who I respected (they were not clinicians) were quite persuasive that my issues were solely mental and that my therapy should be to become more laid back, reduce stress, and learn to "take it easy." Even my earliest doctors discouraged me from ruminating on my symptoms and instructed me to accept them. I learned to deny my own experiences and pain, and this was a huge mistake.

4. *I have learned the necessity of managing my insurance approval process.*

I have been on restrictive policies with various HMOs, which has made the approval process difficult. Still, with enough attention, I have been able to see whom I need. Securing adequate insurance coverage for special procedures and medications has brought its own set of complications. In my experience, insurance providers have denied such coverage mainly for two reasons: there are limitations in regards to contracted providers (doctors or hospitals) and there are limitations for coverage of a given procedure or drug. These limitations are significant but I overcame them by emphasizing medical necessity and supplying the insurers with my diagnosis, case history, and the course of procedures and medications employed. This is how I won my appeals. While my insurance policy may not have allowed the use of a given service or product, the clinical data clearly demonstrated the requested services were the best course of action for my health. The insurance appeal process took effort and time and required my doctor to talk with the insurer's medical director. This was key: getting my doctor on board and committed to taking my case to the insurer. I also spent hours on the phone, drove thousands of miles, spoke with fellow patients, interviewed many doctors, and talked with pharmaceutical companies and reps in order to get what I needed.

5. I have been guilty of believing that I had no choice but to put up with the physical and emotional pain of Crohn's.

I did not realize that I could try to make things better. I have since learned to ask, "Can I influence my own health, or help to make myself better?" I have learned there are new treatments under development and better-trained physicians with more creative ideas. I can also build better health by working with my mind, body, and emotions. I do not have to be a victim anymore.

6. *Crohn's disease left me feeling embarrassed and humiliated, but I do not need to feel this way.*

There is something about Crohn's disease that is particularly odiferous. Having others know of my bowel pain, vomiting, gas, diarrhea, constipation, anxiety, anger, resections, surgeries, procedures, fissures, or fistulas is crappy. I have felt humiliated and ashamed because I was ill. I grew up in a culture that said being ill was a sign of weakness. My family and culture taught me to suck it up, work through distress, and if I did not, I was weak and puny. I went to school or work unless I was completely incapacitated. My embarrassment or humiliation are not useful and I have learned to focus on taking care of myself while realizing that other people are mostly empathetic and supportive of my predicament.

7. *I have learned to stop being afraid to go to the doctor.*

I had a long-time fear that my doctor would give me bad news. I believe some of the delay in my diagnosis was my concern that eventually my doctor would discover a catastrophic disease. I did not want to hear bad news from my doctor and if I avoided my doctor, I would be okay. This ridiculous type of thinking resulted in delaying my care and only created more problems. By going to the doctor, I can get the facts and then can make decisions. Most of the time, my doctor tells me things are stable or I need to make some small adjustments. Occasionally, I might find I need something more extensive like a surgery but I know that by finding issues earlier, I am in the best position to improve.

8. *There are times I have not been forthright with my doctor because I*

felt I was letting him down when my symptoms did not respond well to his treatment.

I see my doctor as a personable, compassionate person and I want to please him. I do not like to come across as whiny and complaining. I need to remember that the purpose of my relationship with my doctor is not to be friends, but instead to work with him to improve my health. I can calmly and clearly tell the doctor that I am in pain. This does not make me weak and frail. He probably feels disappointed with this news but telling him I am "not that bad" when I feel poorly is not acceptable. I need to communicate the truth each time we speak. The fact that I might want to please him is understandable, but our relationship must be one of forthright communications, including giving him bad news when necessary.

9. *Sometimes my doctor has intimidated me.*

I have seen him as someone who is smarter, brighter, or richer than I am; someone who has command over me. I grew up in a family where being a doctor was considered an exceptional profession. A doctor has 10+ years of college experience and training. Yet, even with this, he is not superior to me as a person. He only has superior knowledge in a certain area. I am still the driver of my own health. I have the choice to accept his specific treatment plan or not. I can be vocal and aggressively pursue his help without fear of retribution. I can tell him about my issues, where I need help, and not worry about his response. Doctors are similar to me in more ways than we are different. It is true that in the doctor's office, he has the authority to take charge but he does not shackle me to his exam room or surgery table. It is my choice to work with my doctor as my ally. By doing so, I stand the best chance of making progress in managing Crohn's disease.

Chapter 2 — Gathering My Healthcare Team

A significant part of managing Crohn's disease is through the efforts of my healthcare professional team. An important part of my healing process was to assimilate a healthcare team that would work closely with me. I have identified the key criteria I look for in building a great medical support team.

My General Practitioner

While specialists frequently manage Crohn's, my regular general physician drives most of my healthcare needs. He is the front line in my treatment, is the most available, and can frequently run interference when needed. When I have been healthy, I rarely think about my physician; however, as a Crohn's patient my medical needs are more extensive. I am regularly in touch with my doctor and my demands are greater as my ailment requires more resources to manage effectively.

It is important that my doctor knows the details of my case. In some practices or in some clinics, I used to meet with various doctors in the practice. This is no longer acceptable and I have to work within my healthcare system to find a physician who will be my major point of contact through all of my care. With Crohn's disease, there are details specific to my case that is best handled by one person. Seeing random doctors is not acceptable because there are details that I might forget to convey, it takes significant time to bring them up to speed, and the doctor cannot effectively treat me without understanding the subtleties of my case and history. It is unfair to both the doctor and me not to have a close, extensive relationship.

I have choices within my health plan and thus picking the right doctor is an option. Picking my doctor was not as easy as shopping for a new TV or an automobile. I could not go to Consumer Reports and find easy-to-read data on the skills, personality, and accessibility of a given doctor. While it might be nice to interview a slate of doctors, I have not found it an option to pepper them with questions. Unlike buying a new car, I cannot take doctors for a road test or kick their tires. Instead, I came up with a list of the most important points to consider in choosing a doctor and proceeded to use that as a template.

I need to trust my doctor and develop a relationship of mutual respect. As I work with my doctor and he manages my issues, there will difficult times for both of us. The treatments may not work, there may be poor communication, or it may be just a bad day for both parties. These types of issues are more likely to be calmly dealt with if there is trust and respect and I feel that my doctor is fully committed to taking care of me even with the trials and tribulations of my disease. This does not mean we will become best friends or talk about personal matters, but it does mean that I am confident in his leadership in my case.

In addition to trust, mutual respect is an important quality I look for in a relationship. Respect is based upon goodwill and interest in the other party. There can be disagreements and potential conflicts but if goodwill and respect are present, I can work through the issues. However, respect and trust are projected in different ways and just because a person *appears* nice and friendly does not mean that I should automatically trust them or that they respect me. There are many thieves and scam artists who have a friendly attitude while taking advantage of people. True respect and trust are deeper than simple friendliness and are based upon a fundamental appreciation and commitment to the welfare of others: valuing others as you would yourself. Respect and trust are born out of actions, not mere words and platitudes, and are shown by how people work with others over the long haul.

I need someone who will listen to my story and ask me many questions. My doctor might be able to diagnose me by looking at lab work, x-rays or imaging studies and he might garner additional information by doing a physical exam. However, he will also collect critical data through detailed questioning. My doctor needs to know what has changed since the last time we met, why I am here today, how my therapy is working, what new symptoms I have, and how they present themselves. My doctor needs to listen to my answers carefully and then ask more questions as needed. Another important point is to assume that something has changed since I last saw my doctor. It is easy to say that I am doing the same as before but Crohn's disease varies a lot and changes are likely since my last visit. While they might be small changes, Crohn's disease ebbs and flows and my doctor needs to evaluate me each time in order to make adjustments.

My doctor needs to have the time and be willing to work with me on my case. Taking me on as a patient is a large commitment and a challenging clinical situation. Crohn's disease and its treatment are time-consuming and frustrating. It will require more of my doctor's time and it may challenge his professional knowledge. I have spoken with my doctor about how I need his help and if he has the time to work with me. When I am in acute pain, my doctor needs to see me right away. I am very fortunate that I have rapid access to my doctor and can see him quickly when I am under great duress. He does not just pass me off to the ER where I will have to retell my whole story and not get the ideal treatment. I have not always had this type of access to doctors and I recognize how important it is when considering a physician. Some physician practices are heavily overbooked and it is a challenge to gain access. This is not their fault, but I have chosen to avoid those practices.

My doctor has connected me to a higher level of care when needed. He has picked up the phone and called my gastroenterologist or surgeon, and with his help, I am able to see them within hours when necessary. In the past, I have had some doctors tell me there are others who may be better equipped to handle my challenging case. That is a fair statement on their part for they know how busy their practice is, how skilled they are in this area, and if they can give me the attention I require.

My doctor is willing to work with me to handle my chronic pain. Pain and nausea are major symptoms of my Crohn's disease and they have limited my ability to be active and productive. Some physicians are very conservative about medications, especially when dealing with pain. Their philosophy is, "the less medication, the better." Pain medications can be addictive, have side effects, and must be monitored depending upon one's state of mind. However, it is important to get adequate relief when needed and not to feel shameful about it. I am certain it is not the intent of any clinician to make a patient suffer and I have learned to speak up when I need relief. I am up front with my doctor about my level of pain, if my pain medications are working, and if I am having side effects. My doctor has been supportive in helping me with pain relief and has been supportive of other non-drug pain therapies as well.

I look for my doctor to give me a good exam each time we meet. I look for the classic "pat-a-pat or dig and push" on my belly, his hands feeling the lymph nodes in my neck or groin, and his examination of my mouth and skin. I consider his "clinical handshake" the sign of a good physician who is looking for anything new and what he can learn from my visit. My blood pressure, temperature, eyes, nose, throat, and chest are part of this process. He does this in addition to talking about my bowels. He is like the sleuth with a magnifying glass as he huddles around me trying to sniff out or view any signs or indications that something is amiss. Through his detective work, he has picked up skin lesions, sinus infections, staph infections, and walking pneumonia—all diagnoses that were unrelated to Crohn's but still an important part of my health. He is equally quick with the needle as it relates to my necessary vaccinations or flu shots. I have always appreciated my doctor's interest in my health and think anyone with a chronic health condition like Crohn's disease needs to work with a clinician who looks at the whole patient with each office visit.

My Gastroenterologist

My gastroenterologist drives the detailed aspects of my case. He makes the decisions on Crohn's medications, the need for various therapies, or surgery. He works closely with my primary care physician to make sure I am receiving good continuity of care. Selecting a gastroenterologist is critical with my difficult and complex case of Crohn's disease. I used the same criteria in choosing a gastroenterologist as I did selecting with my general practitioner, but added in some additional skills that were important to me.

I have received at least fifty endoscopies or colonoscopies with six different physicians. I was sedated with versed and fentanyl or propofol for years but required a more general anesthesia for my complex push enteroscopies, ERCP's and balloon dilatations. This was because I became intolerant to propofol that gave me a high fever and rash and my procedures would run two hours or longer. All of the physicians were competent and skillful in their technique but due to my unusual anatomy and complex upper GI strictures, there were times they referred me to other doctors for these procedures. I talked with various physicians and they were able to recommend the "best scope person" for complex cases. For my routine procedures that were straightforward, all of my physicians were able to "scope me." However, my complex procedures with a diseased bowel and significant strictures and hard-to-reach locations required a higher level of skill. For my challenging procedures, including a double balloon push enteroscopy, I searched out a more skilled gastroenterologist who had dealt with these types of cases or used this type of special equipment. Even so, one of my upper endoscopies resulted in a bowel perforation and a major surgery. This procedure was risky and I do not fault the physician, as I knew of the likelihood of complications as we were attempting to dilate the bowel. Even with this perforation, my medical team was able to perform a successful surgical recovery.

My doctors created a detailed treatment plan for my case. I wanted to understand my treatment plan and the different steps in the process. Knowing the details and the ideas behind the treatment plan was important to me; my gastroenterologists shared this information and we talked about it. I was not interested in simply taking the prescribed medications and hoping for the best. I wanted things explained and looked forward to hearing the doctor describe his thinking process and how best to proceed. He would tell me he was going to put me on a given medication, reevaluate me in six months, and then make adjustments if necessary. If we did not get good results, we would consider using another class of drugs and then trial it for another period.

Earlier in my treatment history, I would not ask for and speak with my doctors about the treatment plan. This contributed to my delay in diagnosis and ineffective treatment because I did not know the timeline and what to expect. In contrast, my knowledge of the plan allows me to be more compliant with my therapy and understand any potential issues. It is like using Google Maps or Mapquest on a road trip: I learn where I am going, how long it will take, where I can stop to rest or eat, and the numbers to call if I have a problem.

I have received several additional referrals to different gastroenterologists when my therapies have failed. My complex and unusual case of Crohn's disease required another level of expertise. The GI physicians who work with me have referred me onto other gastroenterologists who specialize in Crohn's disease and limit most of their practice to Crohn's patients. I use my local gastroenterologist for my regular care but use a Crohn's specialist for new and novel approaches to the disease. I would first make my own gastroenterologist aware that I would like him to be more aggressive with my care in order to get better results and if that did not work, he would give me a referral.

It took me five years to realize that I needed another more specialized physician beyond my local gastroenterologist. I have recently learned to use my common sense and evaluate how I am doing with my ailment. If things are not improving and I feel I have exhausted all of the local medical opportunities, then I need to move forward with finding someone who can better assist me with my care. I learned there are different levels of expertise in the area of Crohn's disease and it was my responsibility to take advantage of this when necessary. Doing nothing or settling for the status quo is not a good decision.

My Nurses

Nurses have not been involved with significant clinical decisions in my care. They do not perform procedures, develop complex protocols, or coordinate my surgeries. However, nurses have taken care of me and significantly helped with my comfort and quality of care. For the nurses who have helped me on the phone, in my home, in the doctor's office, in the emergency room, and in the hospital, I am deeply and profoundly appreciative of their efforts. In addition, for any of my whining and complaining and not being appreciative of their efforts, I am sorry. My nurses have been cheerful, optimistic, and genuinely interested in my well-being. They have done their best under challenging circumstances.

I hope that patients who are treated by a nurse will take a few minutes and thank them for their efforts. Writing them a card or sending them some flowers would be a great idea. While nurses may not make the big decisions, they help implement my plan of care as laid out by my doctors. They also supply me with mental and emotional treatment with their kind words, thoughtfulness and cheerfulness, which is an outstanding form of medication. The nurses I worked with are real heroes. I hope they realize that patients like me could not have improved without their help. I extend my heartfelt gratitude and thanks for the wonderful work they do.

Finally, I want to express my sincere gratitude and appreciation for all of the many health care professionals who have helped me over the years. For the most part, they have been patient, kind, skilled and have gone beyond their regular schedules and duties to make a difference in my life. For all of their efforts both in the past and in the future, I am deeply indebted.

Chapter 3 — Finding Personal Support

My personal support team encompasses family, friends, colleagues at work, support groups, and others. I interact with these people on a regular basis and these relationships are a useful and significant part of my healing process. Over the years, I have grown to understand how my relationships can improve my health or make things worse.

I have learned to talk with others about my ailment. Sometimes I am confounded about how to speak with others about Crohn's disease. I do not understand all the technical aspects or science behind my ailment, am embarrassed to talk about it, am uncertain how much others want to know, and do not like to be known as an ill person. I have overcome my ignorance of Crohn's by studying the science behind the disease, talking with doctors, nurses, and reading extensively.

I am also better at managing my embarrassment about Crohn's disease. The genesis of this embarrassment was my humiliation about having a "bowel" disease and acknowledging to others that I am ill. I have learned that I do not need to go into graphic detail about my symptoms and instead I can talk about the nature of an autoimmune disease and the science. While I do not like labeling myself as an ill person, I have addressed that issue by recognizing that most people have some type of chronic problem. For some it might be a physical illness while others might suffer from excessive anger, fear, frustration, or guilt, or have a difficult time managing disappointment and loss. Still others might have a more significant psychological pathology like depression. I recognize that illness is part of the human condition and affects all people at some point in life. The thought that I am not alone with an affliction allows me to accept my condition with more grace.

I also like to be courteous and respectful to people who are interested in knowing how I am doing. They are showing concern about my welfare and their request deserves a polite and kind response. I always thank others for their concern and while my privacy is important, I want to show respect to the thoughtful people who think enough to ask about me.

When people ask me about my disease or how I am doing, I usually say, "I have an autoimmune disorder like arthritis but my ailment creates chronic inflammation in the GI tract." If pressed further, I follow up by saying, "This inflammation can significant symptoms like pain and internal bleeding and when severe, it can require me to take time off work." I will sometimes add, "This lifelong ailment does need medication and some patients eventually need surgery." If they want to ask about my detailed symptoms, I can share this information but I generally do not do this upfront.

When I am acutely ill, I might need to address my health with others in a different way. When I am going through a flare or having a particularly bad day, it is difficult for me to act as thoughtful and upbeat as I normally would. While I do not like to admit to others that I feel terrible or am having a tough day, I think it is important to say something to those who are close to me. I could wear a placard that says "Danger: Crohn's Flare" or "Beware of my Irritated Bowels" but my attempt at a joke will not likely be well received. My confession of illness is not my attempt to gain empathy, attention, or get out of my responsibilities. I tell my close friends and family that I am in distress because a significant flare or pain will be noticeable. If I say nothing, they might observe that I am quiet, moody, or irritated. Unless others know my situation, they may incorrectly assume I am upset at them or upset about an unrelated issue. Thus, I am upfront about my health when needed.

Feeling poorly does not give me license to take my pain out on others or exhibit bad behavior. My distress is not a result of anything they have done. If I am unable to control my mood swings associated with Crohn's, then I will isolate myself from others. This requires self-control and effort but the result is that I am more kind and thoughtful to those close to me.

I have learned to speak to my colleagues and my manager at work about Crohn's issues. In the workplace, having a chronic disease is common. I know others who have diabetes, heart disease, back problems, asthma, or migraines. Still others have bad reactions to life processes like pregnancy or menstruation. With few exceptions, it is not required for an employee to disclose the state of their health to their employer unless it would directly affect their ability to do the job.

When speaking about Crohn's disease with my employer, I

consider three main issues. The first is, am I well enough to do my work? If I cannot perform my job functions, I go home. Even if my manager cannot see any obvious outward signs of my distress, my illness is affecting the quality of my work. It is not fair to the business, my coworkers, or our customers if I work while handicapped. My productivity is down, I am likely to be unpleasant, and others may assume I am lazy or slow rather that ill. However, by telling others that I am ill, I identify the reason for my performance and take the responsibility to leave work until I improve.

I have wondered what my boss or HR thinks about my chronic ailment and my need for time off during a flare. I remind myself that it is normal and reasonable to expect workers to need time off because of illness, surgery, emergencies at home, or needing to care for kids or loved ones. I do not hang my head in shame or see myself as "letting others down" because I cannot fulfill my normal obligations from time to time. Putting myself down will only increase my mental consternation and physical distress.

However, I can improve my relationship with my manager or colleagues impacted by my absenteeism. When I am well, I need to become a real asset for my company. I try to fully engage in my work, be a great addition to the team, and add real value to the company by being as efficient and productive as possible. Good workers are an important asset for any company and while the boss may not like absences, he will respect anyone doing an outstanding job. As I commit to my work, he will see me as a person of integrity and will be interested in my welfare. My best guarantee to maintain a good relationship with my company is to be the best possible employee. This commitment will endear me to the company and bring me personal satisfaction that comes from doing a great job.

I have worried about my health or excessive absenteeism affecting the viability of my job. Can my manager fire me because of my attendance record due to Crohn's disease? While I cannot guarantee this will not happen, I have never seen someone directly fired due to illness. If I were dismissed due to health issues, I would consult the HR department or an attorney if necessary.   However, by being a highly productive employee, my manager is more likely to support me in my times of need. Furthermore, as I take better care of myself each day—getting the best medical care, finding ways to manage my psychological distress, developing more joy and meaning in my life—my ailment can be better managed and I will be more productive with less absenteeism.

My family and friends are an invaluable part of my healing process. Their most healing attributes are friendship, kindness, patience, and thoughtfulness. They boost my sense of well being, bring a smile to my face, make me laugh, share wonderful ideas, and give true meaning to my life. Having good people around me is wonderful medicine. They invoke my deepest appreciation and gratitude with their efforts and this becomes a continual source of healing in my life. I cherish these relationships.

On the other hand, my health is negatively affected by challenging and difficult relationships filled with anger, frustration, guilt, or fear. Difficult relationships sap my energy, fuel intense irritation, and cause my gut to cramp and spasm in biting pain. My negative responses to various relationships have slowed my healing process, exacerbated my symptoms, and caused me to lose weight and have sleepless nights. Finding ways to heal these difficult relationships and manage my departments of anger, fear, and guilt is a critical part of my healing program. I will write about this in more depth later in this book.

Through the computer and various organizations, I have met a new "family" of fellow Crohn's patients. Many Crohn's patients view online forums, participate in posting boards, read about the experiences of others, and eventually meet other patients. There is also a robust national organization, CCFA that has created various support groups in many local communities. These types of interactions help me understand that others are living with this complex ailment and I can learn from them too. The Crohn's community is very courteous and thoughtful both online and in person. Most people recognize that Crohn's disease is serious and thus the overall tone of interactions is generally supportive and kind. Finding others who can directly relate to my issues has been useful to my understanding and healing.

When I have a difficult time with Crohn's, I do not want to obsess about it. I need to be careful that I do not speak excessively about my problems. My obsessive attention on my ailment can *"make a bad thing worse"* because as I focus on my worries and gloom, I generate even more pain and discomfort. Talking at length about my problems with Crohn's can leave me tired and drained. The more I dwell on issues without resolving anything, the worse I feel. This realization initially surprised me because I learned as a child that talking about something makes it better. What my family did not tell me was that talking things through is helpful *only* if I acknowledge the issue but then talk about solutions. Simply rehashing the problem does not help. If I dwell on my problems with no constructive solutions, I relive the pain and become more frustrated and upset.

When I have gone to certain Crohn's meetings or participated in Crohn's postings online, sometimes I have walked away feeling worse. Why? Once again, I made the mistake of talking and listening to many stories of angst with no solutions. I focused on what was not working versus where others or I had made progress. Focusing on pain, discomfort, failed therapy, difficult surgeries, or endless trips to the bathroom is a recipe for disaster. However, talking about solutions and better ways to manage the physical, emotional, and mental issues is healthy. While it is okay to share difficult experiences in a group, I need to complement this with new ideas and strategies that focus on healing.

I have heard many people speak of their disasters with Crohn's and it can be frightening. Being fearful and angry is a reasonable short-term response to a recent flare, surgery, constant pain, unanswered questions about the progressive nature of this disease, and worries about what is going to happen in the future. However, I have scared myself unnecessarily by my own fanciful thinking and listening to the litany of disasters that other people have experienced. A bad experience is a possibility but letting my mind contemplate a worst-case scenario destroys my health by increasing my anger and fear. As I listen to the bad stories of others, my own mind can sometimes think this will happen to me, even if it is not likely.

For example, I remember reading internet board discussions about Versed, a common drug used in colonoscopies and endoscopies. I have taken Versed over fifty times with no issues. However, on the internet boards, many people complained of problems with the drug and warned to avoid it all costs. These people need to find alternative drugs to use—I too have bad reactions to certain drugs—but for most people, taking Versed is safe. There seems to be an allure for people to speak of their bad drugs, surgeries, nurses, doctors or hospitals and the nasty details of pain and suffering. It is like the weatherman spending all his time talking about the bad weather somewhere in the country versus the great weather nearby. I do not want to minimize that bad things happen, but the truth is I tend to bump along with good days and a few bad days but nothing very dramatic either way. I have enough challenges to think about without drumming up more disasters via my own speculations. When I focus on all that could go wrong, I feel worse and cut myself off from the healing energies and stories that improve my health. I will delve further into catastrophic beliefs in a later chapter.

I have to be careful about misinformation. Some of this is based upon misinterpreting information or not taking the time to check the facts. For example, there is a lot of discussion about drug side effects and cancers associated with Crohn's disease. Sorting this out is a complex process. I learned to check out information with a specialist on this subject. My own physicians have not always been able to answer my questions but they have referred me to others who can. In working with Crohn's I need to make sure that I have the facts; I do not want to rely on innuendo, speculation, or hearsay.

The most important relationship that is critical to my healing process is the relationship I have with myself. Nobody has as much of an impact on me as I do. I can take charge of my healthcare and work with various professionals in order to maximize therapy.

I can explore new options to help my condition while working with my mental, emotional, and spiritual self to nurture and bring forth healing energies. I can treat myself with kindness, thoughtfulness, patience, and gratitude to help reduce my internal inflammatory mental and emotional processes. Conversely, I need to be aware that my anger, fear, doubt, worry, and guilt along with non-compliance with my healthcare regime can seriously damage my health and lead to more suffering and pain. My disgust at my own body and resentment in how it is functioning will only bring more problems. How I respond to the pain and aggravation of Crohn's disease is critical to improving my health. I will write about these points later in this book.

Chapter 4 — Managing Crohn's — Pills, Potions, Diet, and More

I have used a variety of healing methods to bring Crohn's disease under control. This chapter delves into how I responded to traditional and alternative methods of therapy.

Drug Therapies

I have not listed a number of commonly used Crohn's drugs because they did not apply to my clinical presentation (in other words, my specific case and location of disease.) Crohn's patients have varying locations of disease and there are different drugs used for different locations, severity, and clinical presentations. I will limit my comments to my own personal experiences with various medications.

My doctors prescribed 6MP (Mercaptopurine) for about eight months and it did not work. I showed no clinical or endoscopic improvement. While taking this drug, I ended up losing 20 pounds due to extreme nausea. I know quite a few people on this fifty-year-old drug who tolerate it well and get a good response; however, it did not work for me.

There is a blood test for this drug that helps determine the optimum dosage because the speed with which patients metabolize drugs varies from person to person. This is useful to maximize the benefits of the drug and minimize the side effects. My blood levels were optimal but the drug was still not useful.

I waited too long to stop taking this drug. 6MP generally takes a few months to create steady state levels in the blood and show its best effects, but I waited much longer. The additional wait time resulted in weight loss, weakness, nausea, time off work, and malaise. I should have been more aggressive with my doctor and described to him how poorly I was feeling so I could have stopped taking it earlier.

After failing 6MP, I tried Methotrexate for four months and experienced the same side effects and no clinical improvement. This time I knew four months is long enough to trial a drug with significant side effects that is not working.

I have been on short bursts of Prednisone (up to sixty days). This drug works well to increase my appetite and give me more energy. However, it does not reduce my overall level of inflammation or the damage to my small bowel, nor does it improve my well-being. My side effects are minimal: some mild jitters, irritability, mild interruption of sleep, and a red glow to my face. There are some long-term negative issues associated with taking Prednisone and if the drug had worked for me, I would have had to balance its short and long-term side effects versus my sense of well being and improvement in symptoms and inflammation. I do know people who have been on Prednisone for thirty or forty years and some of these patients did develop long-term side effects, but for them the benefits outweighed the costs. If you are considering taking Prednisone, this is a discussion to have with your doctor.

I was on Remicade/Infliximab for more than six years. Unlike 6MP, I experienced no side effects from this drug, but also no progress: the drug did not work for me. However, it was the best technology available and the assumption was that something is better than nothing. The doctors did all they could to make it work, but my Crohn's disease remained out of control. During this time, I had two major surgeries due to severe stricturing. While I did not respond to the drug, there were no better options to consider at that time.

A doctor can monitor Remicade through blood testing and in my case; he doubled the dosage because I did not achieve the optimal levels with the normal dose. This still did not help. My doctors then tested me for antibodies to Remicade, which, if positive, could affect its efficacy, and the results were negative.

My doctors considered me a possible candidate for either Humera or Cimzia (in the same class of drugs as Remicade.) However, because I never responded to Remicade and had no antibodies to it, my clinicians felt this was not a worthwhile option. The scientific literature is not clear if switching within the same class of drugs is beneficial if the patient has never responded to that class of drugs. This is a rather complex situation and the data is ever changing as researchers publish new studies. In my case, my doctors chose to move me to another class of drugs and not trial me on Humera or Cimzia.

My doctor then prescribed Stelara: a drug with a different

mode of action than Remicade, Humera, or Cimzia. This drug is currently in late-stage clinical trials and the results are promising. Two publications indicate it may help refractory Crohn's patients like me. It is too early to say how I will respond clinically but thus far, I have experienced no side effects with the medication after one year of use.

My issues with pain management. Finding the best way to manage pain is an important part of Crohn's therapy and while there are a number of pain options to consider, I will focus here on drug therapy. I have been fortunate to respond well to Tylenol (acetaminophen). There are times I take Tylenol for days at a time. There is a lot written about possibly overdosing on Tylenol and I use caution in regards to the daily dose limitations. During times when Tylenol is not strong enough, I take narcotic medications like Hydrocodone or Dilaudid.

I would rather not take drugs at all, especially pain medication. However, the disability I experience from out-of-control pain is much more damaging than the possible side effects. It is hard to work effectively, have a pleasant disposition, or be interested in life when I am in acute pain. I do not have to be pain-free, but the pain should not be overwhelming. For the nastier types of pain such as an inflamed bowel, taking some medication allows me to work a normal day. I find no value in needless suffering. I have worked with my doctor to create a pain program and use the minimum amount of pain medication to gain relief. In addition, I explored other pain options including acupuncture, meditation, and biofeedback, and they helped for mild but not severe pain.

Vitamin B12 deficiency is a common form of vitamin loss associated with Crohn's disease. This is usually caused by the loss of absorption of vitamin B12 in the terminal ilium due to tissue damage or loss. This is treatable by oral ingestion or injection of vitamin B12 depending upon how well the patient responds. My physicians monitor my level of the vitamin B12 with a simple blood test and I have been able to manage my levels with an oral pill.

I have had significant iron-deficient anemia for twenty years and take regular supplementation. Iron deficiency was an early indicator that something was wrong with me although it took years to track down the cause. It showed up as low iron, hemoglobin, and ferritin levels. My doctors focused on my hemoglobin levels that became dangerously low at one point and I required a transfusion.

My doctors placed me on iron pills and I took them for three years. While taking the iron pills did mildly help with my anemia, I never recovered from the deficiency. The iron pills also caused severe abdominal pain. I had a great deal of inflammation in my duodenum and adding iron made it worse. I chose to suffer needlessly from this extra pain when I should have talked with my doctor. It took hospitalization and a blood transfusion for my doctor and me to realize more needed to be done. At that point, my doctor referred me to a hematologist who administered IV iron and I have been on this therapy for eight years with good success. The iron infusions give me more energy, strength, and mental clarity. This experience reminded me to be more aggressive when my therapy is failing.

From this experience, I also learned that people have

different "normal" levels of hemoglobin or iron. My normal hemoglobin levels (a partial indicator of my iron status) are higher than the regular normal range for blood testing. My doctors were concerned when my levels were well below the normal range but they paid little attention when it was near normal. However, my hematologist determined that when given sufficient iron, my normal hemoglobin levels are at the high end of normal and thus the low end of normal is too low for me. The point is, people have different normal ranges and a good hematologist or physician can best determine how to create the optimal level for the patient. By working closely with my doctor, we optimized my therapy and it made a big difference in how I felt.

My doctors routinely tested me for vitamin D levels and they were low. Oral supplements pushed my values into the normal range. There is some evidence that adequate vitamin D levels are important to manage Crohn's disease. I do not understand the science behind how vitamin D levels influence Crohn's, but my doctors feel it is helpful in treating the disease.

My doctors placed me on long-term antibiotic therapy. Within six months of my second major bowel surgery, I was feeling poorly, had significant upper GI belching, nausea, and a loss of appetite. I happened to develop a sinus infection so my doctor placed me on antibiotics, and noted it dramatically improved my nausea and increased my appetite. After completing my course of antibiotics, my symptoms of nausea, belching, and loss of appetite returned. Several months later, I had another sinus infection and the results were the same: taking the antibiotics cured my sinus infection and helped with my appetite and nausea.

I told my IBD specialist and he thought that I might have small bowel overgrowth. He tested me for bacterial overgrowth and the results came back negative. My doctor said the test for small bowel overgrowth is not always reliable so we tried the antibiotics again, for the third time, and my belching and nausea went away, and my appetite increased. Based upon this, he placed me on low dose antibiotics, 25% of the normal daily dose, and I remained at that dosage until my next surgery five years later. I had no side effects from the antibiotics.

This is a great example of how I have learned to listen to my body. I could tell that I went from feeling poorly to feeling great while on antibiotics and we tested this three different times. Based upon this information, my doctor chose to use the antibiotics even though the small bowel overgrowth testing was negative. My body was telling me about a problem and it was showing me the solution. I was also trialed on probiotics, which sounded like a great option in lieu of antibiotics. I tried many different formulations over several months but they did not help. This is most likely because my issues were mostly upper GI that is an area not that sensitive to the use of probiotics.

As a final point to this story, my surgeon removed a piece of diseased bowel in my next major surgery. When my surgeon removed this piece of bowel, I no longer needed the antibiotics. We concluded this piece of diseased bowel was the site of the small bowel overgrowth and stasis.

There is a lot of individual variability when it comes to responsiveness of Crohn's patients to medications. This is influenced by the location and the severity of the diseased tissue and other issues that clinicians do not understand. Thus, someone else might respond to a medication and I will not. I have to work closely with my health care provider and evaluate various medications in order to determine the ones that are best for me. I cannot predict what will work; I have to trial the drug to be certain. Some drugs gave me no side effects while others gave me significant problems. It is common that some medications require a brief period of adjustment and there may be some short-term side effects before the body adjusts. I have learned that after a reasonable amount of time, I should speak with my doctor and decide if I should continue the therapy. I do not need to suffer medication side effects that have no value.

I have been guilty of talking and thinking about getting off my medication. My thought process has been that getting off medication is good and should be the goal. I have learned to understand that medications help me to feel better and I should consider them a blessing and not a curse. Living with Crohn's disease eighty years ago would have been a nightmare with little medical options and I likely would not have survived. Some doctors have spoken to me about the common issue of patients not being compliant with their treatment plans, including medications. It seems a shame to pay a lot of money for the best medical advice but then refuse to follow it. I personally know some patients whose disease has flared up when they took themselves off their medication. While medication does not guarantee the absence of active disease, it gives me the best chance for success.

I have made the mistake of not taking my medication regularly. This is especially true when I am feeling well. By taking medication regularly, I create a therapeutic steady state level of the drug in my system and this constant level of drug is critical. If I am erratic in taking the drug, the level in my blood drops and it might be insufficient to be effective. I need to take the drug as prescribed to get the right levels. There are days, weeks, or months when I might feel good and the disease has somewhat faded into the background of my awareness and I slip back into my old patterns of behavior. Although it is remotely possible that my ailment might fade away for the rest of my life, this is not likely, and eventually it will make itself known again when it comes roaring back for an unexpected visit. While taking medication regularly does not guarantee a permanent remission, it certainly can slow down the likelihood of flares, increase my level of comfort, and help prevent further internal scarring and inflammation. Taking medication is a top priority of my daily routine and is critical if I hope to have the best possible results.

I have been afraid and concerned about taking medication. I felt it was not "natural" and therefore not good for me. I believed that natural was better and I could heal from the foods I eat and the water I drink. I have thought that fabricated items are bad although they are an integral part of my life and the lives of others. I know many cardiac, diabetic, and cancer patients whose lives have either improved or been extended by the use of medications. Man has also developed and optimized many of the foods I eat to contain the best nutrient value. Man has chosen the best possible seeds, livestock, or even algae and fungi to breed or grow for human consumption and this has improved the quality of life for many.

As man attempts to create better options in therapies and healthcare, there are certain risks or possible side effects. I need to evaluate the risks versus benefits and take the medication as prescribed if I determine it adds value to my life. *I have learned to take this one step further and consider my medication to be my friend versus some monster.* As I open the medicine cabinet in the morning and bring out my meds, I say a thank you for its presence in my life. I do not see it as a poison but instead as a gift. Medication does not rebuild worn-out bowel. By itself, it has no real power—the true healer is the intelligence in my body. However, my medication is a catalyst to help my body return to equilibrium. It is the "boost" my body needs. I am fortunate to live in a time when health is a priority for society and medications and other medical interventions are available.

Diet

I started eating "health food" when I was in high school and never stopped. I was a vegetarian for many years and have always eaten highly nutritious food. Over the years as my Crohn's disease has waxed and waned, I have tried to change my diet but have had no success in bringing on remission. During times when I am feeling particularly puny, I have found that eating easy-to-digest foods can help. I create the most nutritious mush diet possible. This was especially important when I was having obstructive symptoms. There are certain hard-to-digest raw foods that have never agreed with me and I avoid these. When I am in the midst of a flare, I use experimentation to change my diet as needed. Certain foods that do not work for me today might work tomorrow; thus I will go back and try foods again that did not agree with me in the past.

My dietary approach to Crohn's is to maximize nutrition and minimize discomfort. Some people think diet is an option to keep their Crohn's disease in remission. I have spoken with a number of people who claim to get a lot of relief on a modified diet. I know others who say they are in full remission by using diet alone, although I cannot verify this. The fact it works for them is something worth exploring. Unfortunately, diet has never controlled my disease.

Regardless of my diet, I never stopped my current treatment program with my health care provider unless he approved it. *Just because I am feeling better does not mean my bowels are healing.* I cannot look inside my intestines and see how I am doing. I cannot scope myself. This is my biggest worry: that I feel better with a therapy or a diet and yet my intestines are still highly inflamed and damage is occurring that could put me in the hospital down the road. Thus if I felt better on any diet or therapy, I want my doctor to scope me to verify that I am healing. I have been surprised in the past when I thought I was doing well only to find out that my bowels were stricturing and I would need another surgery soon.

I did try three months of an elemental diet for Crohn's disease; it tasted awful, and did not work. I was always hungry, it was expensive, and my insurance carrier was reticent to cover it. I gave up this diet when I did not feel better and the tenderness in my gut did not improve.

Elaine Gottschall's Specific Carbohydrate Diet is another diet I tried for a few months. I have met a number of people who have worked with this diet and felt they got good results. I read the book and tried the diet but it did not reduce my active inflammation. I also found the diet high in fat with its use of nuts and oils. My diet requires low fat levels due to complications associated with Crohn's disease and some previous damage done to my pancreas. This type of high-fat diet elevated my blood lipid levels and created problems with my liver and pancreatic enzymes. I was hopeful this diet would work but after a reasonable trail period, I stopped. I also used a similar diet, the Paleo diet, and it too was not helpful.

I used a baby food diet for four years as I experienced obstructive symptoms between major surgeries. I was walking through a grocery store, noticed a sale on baby food, and was intrigued with the variety of foods. They had no preservatives, were low fat, and contained fruits and vegetables. I stocked up and that was the beginning of my "baby food period." I enjoyed the flavors and the huge variety. My baby food diet did not put me into remission but it did help keep my weight on with a reasonably balanced diet. It was also convenient because I could go almost anywhere and buy the food. I used to clean out store shelves when there was a big sale and they had my favorite varieties. This diet stopped when I had another major surgery and could go back to eating more solid foods.

During one flare up period, I was starving. I dropped to 140 pounds (and I am six feet tall!) I was having a seriously difficult time walking, my fatigue was severe, and I had no stamina. My doctor decided to place me on TPN (Total Parenteral Nutrition) for eight months. This is a treatment where all of your nutrients are fed through a tube directly into your blood; thus, your gastro system is not used at all for food. It worked like magic. I gained weight and was able to work a regular day. The pharmacy sent my IV "food" bags to my home and a nurse trained me to clean the entry site in my arm. The hospital placed a PICC line in my arm. I had no infections or complications on TPN, was able to keep the site clean and dry, and became very comfortable setting up my daily dosage. I was able to drink water daily but I got my nutrition via an IV line. I ran my IV during the day and had a portable carrying case that went over my shoulder so I could drive, walk, go to work and do everything but swim.

My experience with TPN was excellent and was a real blessing. If I did not have TPN available, I would have ended up in a long-term hospital stay. Keeping the lines clean and open was a key part of PICC line maintenance. TPN is not an ideal long-term solution although I have read about people who have been on this for years with good results. For me it was a great way to settle down my gut, give me much-needed nutrition, and allow my body to gain strength so I could move forward with my life.

At another time, I lived with a blenderized diet for years. I developed severe strictures and partial debilitating obstructions that required many trips to the emergency room. One day, I was walking through a Costco store and saw a man demonstrating blenders. He was throwing fruits and vegetables into a blender and it came out completely smooth. He was also able to make hot soups, ice cream and various flours from different grains. I thought *This might be a machine to use with my strictures when I cannot eat regular food.*

I used this blender every day for five years and it allowed me to push back a needed surgery by at least four years. Initially I used to make 1-2 quarts every morning with a combination of protein powders, fruits, dried fruits, and various milks like almond, soy, lactose-free and coconut. I would vary the recipes but made a highly nutritious drink of 1000 calories per day. I bought some pint and quart containers and my doctor wrote a prescription that allowed me to take my liquid diet onto an airplane.

While the diet does not sound exciting, I could also cook certain meats and vegetables just as I normally would but finish by throwing it all in a blender. I made a blenderized breakfast and dinner. My weight remained stable, I had no obstructive issues, and my blood work was within normal limits. This type of blenderized eating was useful to get adequate calories and nutrition with less pain due to my obstructive symptoms. While I recently had another major surgery that allows me to eat normally, I would consider using the blenderized eating option in the future if needed.

I was concerned about the lack of nutrients in my blood due to malabsorption associated with surgeries and Crohn's disease. I worried that taking supplements and simply hoping they were being absorbed was not a good approach, so I had special testing done to look for malabsorption, my levels of key nutrients, and food allergens. These esoteric tests and traditional tests gave me confidence that I was getting adequate nutritional intake and absorption. We also tested for some esoteric metabolic compounds that we quantified by blood testing in a number of specialty laboratories. Based upon these results, my healthcare team was reassured that my levels were adequate. Armed with this data, I do not have to worry about taking vitamins, minerals, and special nutrients. The test results reassured me that all is in order.

I worked with both a Chinese herbologist and an Ayruvedic physician for a number of years evaluating various combinations of herbs to help placate my active Crohn's disease. I enjoyed watching these specialty physicians come up with unusual mixtures of herbal medicine and learning about the knowledge behind the treatments and the impact they might have on my various imbalances and doshas. I followed their advice and while these treatments were pleasant, I did not note any improvement in my Crohn's disease.

Meditation, Acupuncture, Reiki, Chiropractic Care & Panchakarma

I tried meditation to improve my emotional and mental health and help with my inflammation. I started practicing meditation as a teenager and continued for over thirty years. I attended many advanced courses and received advanced techniques. Meditation helped create a strong experience of restfulness, energy, and increased peacefulness. However, this process was not able to reduce my gut inflammation or spasms or help me better manage other various dysfunctional mental and emotional issues.

I had many panchakarma treatments (including abhyanga, shirodhara and basti) that left me feeling refreshed and more enlivened. These treatments calmed me down and reduced my overall irritation but did not put me in remission and their effects quickly wore off.

I have taken and completed the first part of Reiki training, and have identified an outstanding acupuncturist whose treatments have some effect on calming down my overactive gut. I have also benefitted from a chiropractor. This particular non-force chiropractor has helped me with pain management; his techniques help me recover from various physical issues like surgery gut spasms. All three of these specialists are helpful for short-term relief.

I have exercised throughout my adult life. This has varied from strenuous exercise with heavy aerobics to light weight lifting to walking. For the last few decades, I have taken a brisk walk of two or three miles at least once per day. Walking helps reduce my pent-up energy and angst while doing great things for my stamina and blood pressure. The resulting stamina has helped me rapidly recover from surgery and appears to aid with my digestion. I also spent time in physical therapy to help manage chronic pain and muscle tension and found it useful.

Dealing with a chronic incurable disease like Crohn's is very complex process and requires multiple approaches. I explored many possible options, read extensively, and noted items that looked interesting or promising. I tried a variety of methods or products and observed how I responded. When taken together, all of these methods have had an impact on my well-being.

I use some of these tools for non-Crohn's related issues. For example, I see my chiropractor not because I have Crohn's but because I enjoy how he works with my body and the feel of his therapeutic touch. My acupuncturist's treatments create a deep sense of quiet and restfulness. Meditation has an overall calming effect and I do enjoy massage treatments as well. The herbs and teas I use are pleasing; walking helps with my blood pressure and stamina.

Putting all of these tools together has allowed me to live better with Crohn's disease and be productive while reducing my discomfort and fatigue. While the improvement to my quality of life might only be 1-2% with some of the above modalities, that to me is a win. I will take any improvement as I try to move closer to the goal of improved health.

Chapter 5 — When Surgery Becomes Necessary

As part of the normal process of Crohn's disease, 70% of patients will need surgery at some point in their life. I have had ten surgeries, including eight abdominal and three major open procedures. When I first considered surgery, I found it a scary nightmarish process. However, the net effect of surgery is that my life significantly improved and I enjoyed many new experiences and opportunities. With one exception, my surgeries enhanced rather than decreased my quality of life.

Making the Decision

The biggest issue associated with my own surgical process was when to do it. While I did have one emergency surgery due to a perforated bowel, all of the other surgeries were elective. I was able to talk with my surgeon and doctor and determine if it was the right time to proceed. In general, I found that I waited too long to have each surgery. For me, the underlying reasons for my major surgeries were debilitating obstructions and pain. In each case, my doctors did not push me to have surgery because they wanted to maintain the integrity of my bowel and I did not tell them how lousy I felt. I was being overly heroic and did not want to complain. In some delusional way, I felt things were not that bad and I could suffer along each day and survive. When I contrast this with how much better I felt after the surgery, I realized how my delay adversely affected my health.

Fear and uncertainty played a strong role in my surgical delay. My thoughts contributed to my delays in having surgery: imagining a surgeon cutting me open, wondering if I would wake up, and worrying that I would be in too much pain. I suffered from disaster-orientated thinking and I learned to handle this by educating myself on the surgery and recovery process. Knowledge is a great antidote to catastrophic thinking. I also found it useful to visualize the entire process in my mind. I visualized a great surgical team made up of good people working hard to create an exceptional result. I saw their commitment and skills and reminded myself that they are experts in what they do and have years of experience to draw upon. Through this visualization and reassurance process, I became more comfortable.

Choosing a surgeon

Through my surgical experiences, I created three key criteria that are important to me in choosing a surgeon. I looked for a surgeon who: 1) would outline his plan for the surgery and my normal course of recovery; 2) had a high level of expertise with working on my type of complex issues; and 3) would answer my detailed questions while understanding the value of mental health in the healing process. I see it as a team effort. My surgeon supplies the surgical skills while I supply the proper physical self-care and important psychological optimism and healthy healing attitude. Our combined efforts lead to the best results.

I like to understand how my surgeons view my case and if they have observed similar issues before. I want to hear about their experiences with patients like me. This gives me a level of confidence and a reasonable idea what to expect. When I was "shopping for surgeons" for my last surgery, I found two surgeons who talked about their surgical plans and shared their experiences and my likely recovery period.

The second issue is competence. All of my surgeons have been competent in their skills, but only a few had many years of experience working with Crohn's patients with a complex history. My last surgery was very complex and involved and when I discussed this with my local surgeons, they readily admitted they did not have extensive experiences with this type of surgery and it would be a challenge for them. I thus searched for and found a surgeon who had extensive experience in these types of cases. The results were exceptional, the recovery quick, and I attribute this to the experience level of my surgeon. Based upon my first-hand knowledge, I recognize that in complex cases having a very specialized surgeon makes a huge difference in both the outcome and the speed of recovery.

My final issue is that I want my surgeon to work and talk with me. I want him to see me as a willing partner in the process who will be highly compliant during the recovery period. I will work on my mental and emotional self to create a harmonious environment of patience, kindness, gratitude, and peace as I heal and recover. These powerful mental and emotional energies are important to true healing and I want my surgeon to recognize their value and see that we are healing both a sick body and an injured mental and emotional self that has suffered years of chronic illness. Not all surgeons have this orientation but I was fortunate to find one and the results were excellent. We were healing my entire self, not just my irritated bowel.

Choosing a hospital and staff

I had surgeries in four different hospitals. The hospitals had a good staff, were competent in their processes, and I had no complications or issues in any of the facilities. However, as part of my preparation for surgery, it was important psychologically to visit each hospital. I was able to observe the check-in process, view the pre-op area, look inside an operating room, view a recovery room, and see the location where I would be staying. The staff was kind enough to show me around and I found seeing the entire setup made the whole idea of surgery less frightening. I noted the staff and the nurses were regular folks just like me. They talked about their commitment to what they did and were very forthcoming in answering my questions. They were efficient and skilled and I came to realize that my anxiety was simply in my head. When I saw with my own eyes the great people who would be part of my care, I felt more relaxed and confident.

I observed there are different levels of sophistication or care at different hospitals. Some of the hospitals had a larger staff, were more responsive, and had more innovative technology available. Some of their procedures seemed to give me better results and their level of patient care and attention was exceptional. At one hospital, while I did not have my own private nurse, it seemed like I did because my nurse was so attentive. I recognize that not all hospitals have the same resources and therefore in a complex medical case like mine, I want to use the higher-end hospitals to get that extra level of care. This is not a critique on any particular hospital but an acknowledgement that there is a difference.

Choosing open versus laparoscopic surgery

I spoke to my surgeon about an open versus a laparoscopic surgery. I read about the wonders of laparoscopic surgery and I had one in the past and enjoyed a speedy recovery time. I felt an open surgery would leave me with more pain and a long recovery time. Today, most surgeons will attempt to do a procedure laproscopically as they understand its benefits. However, in my case, the surgery was complex and my surgeon said he could attempt it laproscopically but it would greatly increase the surgery time. This procedure would force him to focus a lot of time on the laparoscopic manipulations versus concentrating on the repair work at hand. He was telling me a laparoscopic procedure would inhibit his ability to do the best job. Thus, I chose the open procedure for my complex case. Issues like adhesions, previous surgeries, location of the disease, and the need to work with complex anatomy all played a role in this decision. Looking back, I went through three major open procedures with great success. While there was pain after the procedure, my clinicians controlled it well, the healing was uneventful, and I got the results I needed.

Not my best surgery

One of my major surgeries did not go well. The surgery itself was uneventful with no complications and I healed when I returned home. However, I did not get the type of relief I expected following the surgery. I limped along for five more years until further stricturing and obstructions resulted in my need for another surgery. During this time, I required hospitalizations, TPN or IV feedings; had significant pain and nausea; was on a liquid diet; and required regular antibiotic use due to bacterial overgrowth. I was anemic, run down, and unable to do my normal activities. I had to exercise with caution, limit my travel, and make other lifestyle adjustments in order to get through the day. I continued to work and my business prospered although I had to take great care with my health. This was a very difficult period for me as my life became limited and restricted. Looking back, I realize that I was learning how to handle adversity and while it was not pleasant, I learned new coping skills that have helped me in all parts of my life. I changed many of my activities and focused on working on my mind and emotions in order to gain better mental control over my situation. I learned to fend off any negative pessimistic and destructive thinking that would make a bad situation worse while appreciating deeply the generosity and support of those around me. I saw myself not as a diseased person but rather a person who has a diseased area in his body. I learned to laugh more, treasure the good moments, and be more accommodating of difficult times. This time of illness was transformative for personal growth and while I would not wish it on anyone, its benefits included forcing me to focus on what was most important while giving me an incentive to develop great mental tools and a healthy perspective on life.

Looking back, I can see now that this unsuccessful surgery was too minimal. My excellent and kind surgeon chose to take a more minimalistic approach to the surgery and while he cleaned up the worst areas, he left behind an area of diseased tissue. One anatomically complex area in the duodenum and adjacent to the ampulla of vater was tightly strictured and impacting my normal pancreatic and biliary flow. Removal of this stricture was complex and it was left untouched. In hindsight, I knew my case was complex and I should have pursued the opinion of an experienced Crohn's surgeon who could have handled this technically difficult surgery and I would have avoided a lot of misery. I learned from this mistake and made sure I addressed all of the diseased areas in the next surgery and the results were outstanding. With the following surgery, I was able to ramp up my daily activities due to an increased level of energy; eliminate antibiotics, pain medication and the need for iron infusions; and could now eat normally. Pursing a surgeon with additional expertise and skills is a wise decision for a difficult case and made a huge difference with me.

I do not blame anyone for my poor surgical results. I am certain my surgeon was as unhappy as I was with the outcome. These things happen—but knowing what I know today, I would be fully committed to making sure my surgeon addressed all of my diseased tissue during the surgery.

Preparing for my surgical stay

My extensive surgeries required a seven- to eight-day hospital stay. I chose to set up my hospital room to be as comfortable as possible. I brought my own pillow and some of my own sheets. I also had my own room and the hospital staff was able to set up another bed for my wife so we could visit and rest together. Other than the daily walks around the nursing station and the occasional visits with friends and family, there is not a whole lot to do. I usually wake up at all kinds of strange hours and while they offer me sleeping and pain medication, there are times I want to stay awake. The entertainment center in my hospital room has historically been weak so I brought along some light reading, an iPod for music, and a video system that I used extensively during my stay. Some nights I listened to music all night to cut down on the buzzing and whirring background noises. These pleasant distractions made for a more comfortable stay and helped pass the time.

Being confident and leaving behind anxiety

Being confident that my recovery will go well is a critical component of my preparation for a hospital stay. With increased confidence, I am much more likely to remain relaxed, experience less pain, heal faster, and sleep better. Thus, I work on my mental attitude as I approach surgery and recovery. I focus on the following points:

My pain will be tolerable and under control. There are many pain medications and spinal block technologies available. I have never been in significant pain while in the hospital. In fact, I have more pain at home with a Crohn's flare or obstruction than post-surgery in a hospital. The staff is extremely concerned about my level of discomfort and they give me what I need to be comfortable. "On a scale of 1-10, what is your pain level?" replaced "Good day" as the refrain of choice for the staff each time they came into my room. The only way I could experience significant pain would be to deny the medication they offer me.

The staff is rooting for me and they cheer for me. They carry around symbolic mental "pom-poms" and applaud me each day. They greet me with a smile, ask what I need, and take pride in their level of care. They nourish me mentally with their kindness and thoughtfulness, and in some strange way I nourish them too by accepting their care, being a compliant patient, and expressing gratitude. Whatever I need or desire, I only ask and they are ready to help. The only downside to all of this great service is that I cannot take it home with me after I leave the hospital!

I will wake up after anesthesia. I have worried about having a bad drug reaction to anesthesia, becoming ill, or not waking up post-surgery. There are no guarantees that reactions will not occur; however, I remind myself that I have had anesthesia over 50 times with surgeries, endoscopies, and colonoscopies and have experienced no issues. The technology behind anesthesia is outstanding and the staff are doing all they can to prevent reactions or other issues. There are medications available if I become nauseated. The anesthesiologist is willing to explain to me his process and during surgery, he is carefully monitoring my vitals and making certain I am in good shape. This allows the rest of the staff to focus on the surgery.

I just say no to horror stories. By going online, talking with people, watching TV, and seeing movies, I have found some situations or fantasy scenes that portray a horror story about hospitals or surgeries. Some of these stories are true and mistakes or unusual circumstances do occur. However, for the vast majority of people and especially those with no extensive complicating factors, there are no problems with surgery and recovery. After my healthcare team reviews my case, they will design a protocol to give me the best possible result. With all of this preparation and medical skill in place, I am in an excellent position to discount or ignore any lingering doubts that can create fear in my mind. Thus, I remind myself to leave the scary mental stories of monsters and disasters to those times when I want to be scared or get a thrill: going to a horror movie, reading a horror novel, or being on an outrageous ride at an amusement park. My fear and anxiety related to disastrous surgical outcomes have no usefulness during my hospital stay and I do not indulge them.

Getting up and going in the hospital

Getting out of bed is a critical part of the healing process. Usually, during my first day post-surgery, I am groggy and other than someone trying to move me with a crowbar, I am busy sleeping off the medication and resting. However, starting with day two, the nursing staff is on me to get moving. This is useful for several reasons.

Walking helps to prevent blood clots and improve my circulation. The staff uses other tools to manage clotting issues like compression leggings (puffy leggings) or various medications but good old-fashioned walking around is invaluable. The staff helps to steady me and then off I go on my journey into the hallways, walks around the nurses' station or to various viewing locations so I can look outside and observe the weather. As I "run" this course, others greet me with their IV poles in hand as they meander about. Walking is also useful because it stimulates my lungs and helps me cough up phlegm and increase my blood oxygen levels. When I return to bed, I might find the nursing staff has left behind the next-best thing to chocolate on my pillow: a brand new plastic device called a Spirometer that I can use to stimulate my lungs while in bed.

My first "serious" trip to the bathroom

After surgery, my bowels go to sleep as a normal part of the healing process. This hibernation period varies depending upon the type of surgery and the patient. The medical staff constantly prods me about my bowel habits and it is clear that the staff is waiting to hear the news that things have begun to "move" again. For those who have taken a child through potty training, the experience is similar. There is a lot of hopeful anticipation and then accolades and praise for a job well done. I half-expected to hear band music and a public announcement on the intercom after this great accomplishment. However, all kidding aside, active bowels are a hallmark moment that says liquids and solid food are just around the corner. This is an acknowledgement that physical healing has taken place and I am moving in the right direction. This generally took 4-5 days after my open surgeries.

My first food

Eating for the first time post-surgery is always an interesting experience for me. It feels different because I have new plumbing in place. My response to food and my digestive process changes over time until my body establishes its new normal. For me, this rapidly occurs over the first few weeks and months and continues for up to one year. My doctors say that my digestion will normalize in a month or two, but they are always wrong and it takes much longer. I am not in pain or necessarily having a tough time but it means that the final healing process takes longer than they told me. I learn to experiment with different foods and find new foods that work best with my new plumbing.

At home

I keep active when I get home. I take walks each day and gradually increase my time. I find this continues to help my lungs and my digestion seems better with walking. I continue to experiment with food; the foods I managed well pre-surgery are not necessarily the ones that work best post-surgery. I focus on high nutrient content in order to give my body the material it needs to heal. This is always a lot of fun as I generally go into surgery with a lot of narrowing's and a restricted liquid diet of mush. It is exciting to come out of surgery and eat real foods that go crunch and do not make me sick.

It always takes me longer to heal than my doctors tell me. While my progress is good and steady, my experience of twinges, aches, fatigue, or pain always takes longer to fully resolve. This is especially true in the first 4-6 weeks. I am not miserable and uncomfortable but I cannot jump back into a normal routine. I learned a lot about patience and taking time to let the healing occur as I watched my big suture line slowly stop draining and become less sensitive. As I accepted this longer timeline, my mind was able to relax and be more confident that things were moving in the right direction.

Thanking my body

I rejoice in how much better I feel after surgery. The same way I give thanks and appreciation to those around me who helped me through my surgical process, I need to give thanks to my body and myself. This may sound bizarre, but it is a critical part of my healing process. I need to recognize what I have accomplished. Surgery is tough for most people and yet I have succeeded. This surgery is going to enhance all parts of my life and affect me in many ways. I give thanks to my body and its intelligent healing properties. It has mended the tissue, grown new cells, and brought life into the healing area. My appreciation of this miraculous feat is a celebration of a miraculous process. I try to make time for a "healing celebration" at home soon after the surgery. While it might not be a four-course meal, it includes the comfort of wonderful family and friends, the chance to give thanks, and the time to note my body's achievement.

I want to preserve my gains and I make a commitment post-surgery to eat highly nutritious foods, drink a lot of water, get enough sleep, and take my medications as prescribed by my doctor. I remain focused on my mental, emotional, and spiritual health and work to manage my own psychological irritations.

I remind myself that I have gone through this successfully and attempt to commit it to memory. Thus, if I need to go through this again in the future, I am creating a memory of success and achievement that I can recall and use in difficult times.

Finally, I let my physician know if anything seems amiss. While I have been fortunate enough to heal after each surgery and procedure, I have noticed a few odd twinges, tweaks or oozing around the surgical site or some other unusual experiences. While not overly concerning, this type of information is important to communicate back to my doctors so they can continue to manage my recovery and help me ward off any unexpected issues.

Thanking the staff and my family

I need to remember that when I go through these procedures, it is affecting my family, friends, surgeon, and the medical staff as well. I could easily slip into the mindset of "woe is me" and focus on all of the troubles and issues I have to deal with, but I need to remember that others are living through this surgery, too, with all its ups and down. The following is a letter I wrote to friends and family after my last surgery while recovering at home. I think this letter summarizes my thoughts on the importance of others in my healing process and the roles they played.

Dear All,

As I am recovering from surgery, I want to pass along a few thoughts and acknowledgements. I am grateful for all of your thoughtfulness, prayers, and best wishes on my behalf. I appreciate all of your efforts in invoking these blessings.

I want to thank both of my daughters, Shanna and Laura, for their efforts while I was hospitalized. Laura was so helpful to Mary Lou (my wife) and me in taking care of our dog Gracie. Gracie became ill while I was in the hospital. Laura and Michael took her from the kennel to the vet, and then they stayed with her in our home while Gracie improved.

I want to thank my daughter Shanna for taking time off work and coming out to visit while I was in the hospital. Her smiling face and cheerfulness were great and I am appreciative of her efforts to keep family and friends informed about my progress. This helped Mary Lou and I keep in touch. I am also thankful that when Shanna arrived, she was able to whisk Mary Lou away from the hospital to the local hotel and stay with her in a nice clean room with good meal service, a comfortable bed, and number of nights of uninterrupted sleep. Mary Lou was exhausted after spending four nights in my room post-surgery with little sleep and food.

Thanks to all of you who were able to visit me in the hospital. My apologies for not being Mr. Personality as you came by but hopefully I was not too crabby. However, I want each of you to know that I am thankful to all who reached out to Mary Lou with their kind words of support, hugs, or taking her downstairs for a cup of tea or a meal in a local restaurant. I have not experienced it, but it must be extremely tiring and difficult to take care of a sick or recovering loved one. (From my perspective, being the patient is easier than being the caregiver!) Mary Lou was beside me and answered my calls when I needed help and she watched over me to make sure my care was 100%. She bathed me, listened to my concerns and she did it with a smile and love in her heart. For me to know that each of you were reaching out to her, supporting her, taking care of her, and visiting with her was the greatest gift that you gave me.

During the first 3-4 nights after surgery, I would wake up many times through the night in a dark room full of blinking lights, the sounds of equipment pumping fluids and the nursing staff moving about the hallways. It would always take me a few seconds to remember where I was. However, I would always look over to the bay window that was about ten feet way and see Mary Lou sleeping there with her quiet rhythmic breathing. For those of you who did not see her sleeping area, she slept in a three-foot wide bay window that looked out on a courtyard. With the help of the nursing staff and some items we brought from home, they were able to build a reasonably soft bed there that she could sleep on each night. For me it was like having a princess resting comfortably a few feet away in this room of blinking lights and different sounds. I enjoyed looking at her and seeing the soft features of her face in the subdued light *and I felt so thankful for her presence. She has always been so gracious to me and she is someone to love and to cherish, in good times and in bad, and in sickness and in health. As I saw her each night, she was and is my "Sleeping Beauty."*

I also want to comment about the medical staff at this medical center. I have spent time in a number of hospitals over the years, and this group was the most attentive, professional and the most skilled that I have ever experienced. The staff truly had my best interest in mind. The hospital even has healing dogs that come into the hospital three times per week and I was fortunate to meet these therapeutic and friendly pets.

I want to mention my gastroenterologist and surgeon. I have been under the care of some excellent doctors and surgeons both here in my hometown and in Los Angeles. Up until a little more than a year ago, I had not met the two doctors who worked with me. However, their combined efforts have been outstanding.

Finally, I have newfound energy and can now eat, for the first time in almost a decade without pain, non-blenderized food with texture, shape, and form. In my first few weeks after surgery, I have grown to appreciate a crispy piece of toast, real chucks of fruit and my new favorite: vegetable soup with real chunks of vegetables. It is an amazing experience! I look forward to the possibility of trying a bean tostada, real oatmeal with texture, and hope to ultimately graduate to a fresh salad. The whole experience of eating solid food is a new one after years of not being able to eat without pain or nausea.

You all have filled my life with continual blessings and I am very grateful.

With love and appreciation, Jim

Chapter 6 — Psychological Help

Following my second major surgery, my appetite was minimal, my pain excessive and my enthusiasm for life was waning. I worked harder on all my regular and alternative therapies. This effort was helpful and for four years I slowly improved and pulled myself back from the 140-pound, six-foot tall exhausted and dismayed person I had become. Some of the key tools that helped during this time were eating blenderized food, dietary adjustments, the daily use of antibiotics, TPN, learning to sleep in a chair, iron infusions, finding a more experienced physician, better pain management, and more extensive use of chiropractic care. Yet my active Crohn's disease and psychological challenges continued unabated and after some time, I noticed myself starting to slip again into the rabbit hole of hopelessness. I attempted to adjust my therapy and with each attempt, I perked up briefly, only to slide back down again. It was like taking one step forward and two steps back. I was just spinning my wheels and slowly digging myself into a deeper hole.

I remember several visits to my gastroenterologist. My doctor told me we had done everything medically possible but if needed, I could get more pain medication. During another visit, I sat with my doctor and we reviewed my most recent blood work. I was told my blood work and weight looked like someone who was starving. My serum protein, albumin, and calcium levels were low and my immunology suggested I had an immune deficiency problem. I could see and count all of my ribs, my face looked hallowed, my skin color was pasty white, and I had little energy or vitality. I was starving nutritionally—and mentally, too. I was devoid of hope and optimism and it was a struggle to get through each day. My trajectory was downhill and I realized I needed other options.

This sense of pending doom got me thinking, "What else can I do?" One day, I awoke with a new approach to my problem. Before I speak about my new idea, I wish to emphasize that I was going to continue using all of my physical tools to heal and look further for better physical options as they became available. If I hurt, I was going to take pain medication, have surgery, and look at other pills, potions, diet, manipulations, and meditations as needed.

My new idea was this: I have a physical body and it functions well, except for part of my digestive system. I have some inflammation in my gut and am unable to absorb nutrients and properly flush away the waste. I had done all that I could physically, yet it was still a problem. I then thought about the massive amount of material I had read over decades on new age thought, including the idea that we are multidimensional beings. We are more than just physical forms: we are also mental, emotional, and spiritual beings, too. While I had read about these ideas and embraced them for years, I never seriously applied them to my treatment of Crohn's disease. In no way had I thought to work with my mental, emotional, and spiritual self to help my physical body to heal. I still approached Crohn's disease as a physical issue and worked with pills, potions, diet, exercise, and a knife to manage it.

Over the next year, I worked to come up with a program of building and creating better health in all parts of myself. I reasoned that if I was truly a combination of physical, mental, emotional and spiritual, I needed to work with all of these aspects, as they are connected. This is evident in a simple example: if I let myself get upset or angry, this causes my stomach to churn or my head to hurt. Thus, my emotional upset must be influencing my physical self. On the other hand, if I became exhausted, my mind does not think clearly. Thus, my physical issues are impacting my mind. It was obvious that the physical, emotional and mental parts of me were connected and influencing each other. I wanted to take advantage of this realization and use it to heal.

The balance of this book is my effort to work with the non-physical parts of myself and create pragmatic healing tools and techniques. It has taken me time to put this program together and it is still a work-in-progress. I realized my mental, spiritual, and emotional makeup has changed very little over decades. The way I react and respond to life today is similar to how I did in my youth. I failed to update my mental and emotional software. I recognized the need to work with my mind and break old habits, deal with mental bodyguards, and discard old worn-out beliefs. This was a major demolition and remodeling job involving my character.

As I have worked with this program, Crohn's disease has not gone away. It has not left behind a "gone fishing" sign. It remains with me and occasionally clamors for attention. I still have a chronic ailment that that is not curable. However, its angry demeanor and irritable nature have acquiesced as I experience less fear and guilt. I have built better health through developing healthy beliefs and increasing my joy, gratitude, and forgiveness. My tissues are clearly happier endoscopically and microscopically then they have been for some time and I attribute this to better physical treatments and to mental work that keeps my mind stronger as I no longer fan my internal flame of irritation and anger.

Building health is not the same as fighting disease. For me, fighting disease involves attacking the main manifestations of the ailment and doing what is necessary through drugs, surgery, or other "emergency" therapies to relieve my symptoms and remove or eliminate the malady. This is especially important in the midst of flare. By comparison, building health is what I do when I wish to fortify myself and create more robustness, power, and vibrancy in all parts of my mental, physical, emotional, and spiritual selves. Both methods are required to manage and live gracefully with Crohn's disease.

I have learned there is more to health than a healthy body. I see people who are remarkable physical specimens with very robust bodies. Yet, some of these same people are chronically angry, depressed or even anxious. This to me is not true health, regardless of the state of their physical bodies. True health is healthiness of mind, body, and spirit.

Sometimes I see the ebbing and flowing of Crohn's disease is like living by a river. Most of the time life by the "river" is good. However, occasionally the river (of inflammation) rises and floods my physiology and mind. I am never exactly sure when this will happen. Even if there have been many years of low water and no floods, it is possible that I will experience another flood of inflammation and a flare. This creates a lot of uncertainty and as a Crohn's patient, I am married to this predicament and need to do what I can to manage the inflammatory floods whenever they come.

For me it is not whether or not the flood (of Crohn's Disease) will come, it is more a matter of when. If the flood comes I can deal with it as an acute situation and bring forth all of the medications, drugs, surgeries, and alternative therapies available. This is attacking the symptoms and the disease. However, there are other things I can do is to prepare for the storm that will come at some point. I can fortify my home, make the walls stronger, raise the house, put in a water pump, and place sandbags around it. I do this by working with my physical, emotional, mental, and spiritual selves. I have fortified the structure of myself to handle these floods with more grace and ease, and less mental inflammation, irritation, and pain.

This is analogous to the story of the three little pigs. I need to be like the third little pig who builds his house with bricks. Even though this requires more effort than the other two pigs that do the minimum amount of work, the payoff for the third pig is obvious when the big bad wolf of Crohn's disease appears. The stability of the house of bricks is the foundation that allows the third pig to keep the wolf (Crohn's) away. I need to be like the smart pig that does all he can to build a structure that will provide more comfort and stability during difficult times. I must build my own "house of bricks" with better tools that nourish and strengthen my physical, emotional, mental, and spiritual selves.

My approaches to healing and building health are real ideas and processes that I have personally tried and worked with. They may not work for all people; others may find different options. For me, this work has created an opportunity for personal growth and a new sense of hope and optimism. I have brought the non-physical—the other three-fourths of myself—into action and have built better health, thus getting a handle on this cruel disease. The following chapters describe my process.

Chapter 7 — Using the Mind for First Aid

There were times my Crohn's disease overwhelmed me. I felt like I hit a wall that was preventing me from having any semblance of a decent day. The trigger might be the steady accumulation of disappointments, or having to spend another day in the bathroom or in bed. Sometimes it would be nonstop pain and nausea or other personal changes. Whatever the reason might be, at times it was too much to bear. Despite doing all the usual things I knew how to do, I felt trapped and helpless by a problem that never seemed to end. I needed something extra—an emergency kit of special mental tools—to get me through these tough passages.

Before I elaborate on this mental tool kit, I must emphasize that it is important to evaluate your current condition to determine if the major problem is an escalation of your medical condition or whether this is just more discouragement and frustration. You want to be certain this is not a critical medical condition that requires the experience of a health care provider. If you feel your current symptoms are significant medical events—for example, if they are causing great physical distress, or you feel uncertain about what to do—this is not the time to delay. Contact your health care provider, dial 911, or go to the emergency room.

I have had 25+ emergency rooms visits associated with Crohn's disease. While most of them were resolved with simple reassurance from medical staff and various procedures, there were three instances when my delay getting help made things worse. For example, I obstructed after eating pistachio nuts while visiting New York City. My pain and vomiting became so extreme that I had to lie down on the sidewalk, in the rain, in the upper westside of Manhattan. (Pistachio nuts are great, but not with a narrowed bowel!) I needed an ambulance ride and a 16-hour hospital stay and workup. I was fortunate that this happened in a large city with great medical care; otherwise, my outcome could have been much worse.

The second event was a perforated small bowel, which brought on pain so intense I could not move. My small bowel perforated during an upper endoscopy and the symptoms did not start until I returned home. The pain came on suddenly and I tried to "grin and bear it" for three hours, thinking it would get better. (Bad decision!) This delay exacerbated my emergency surgical recovery due to bacterial contamination.

My third occurrence was another obstructive event after a Christmas dinner that was delicious but too much roughage for a narrowed gut. I delayed this trip to the ER until extreme nausea, vomiting, pain, and the threat of a 911 call by my wife drove me there.

In each of these three cases, the event was significant because it came on suddenly, I was overwhelmed, and was unable to stand or walk. In hindsight, these events were notably out of the ordinary and there were obvious signs that something was amiss. Nevertheless, in each case, I delayed my trip to the ER by a number of hours as I tried to suck it up, which was a serious mistake. My advice is to seek medical help quickly when you are experiencing uncontrollable medical symptoms. While the ER staff managed my cases, I endured more pain and a higher possibility of complications than was necessary.

Prescription medicine for psychological pain

If you are reasonably certain that there is no medical emergency, then read on—the rest of this chapter focuses on tools I use to more effectively manage my thinking and mood.

While I am not a prescribing physician, I am familiar with many medications used to manage acute and chronic mental distress: drugs such as anxiolytics, anti-depressants, and benzodiazepines. I have taken both short- and long-acting medications to give some relief to my mental angst; I also evaluated and ingested various herbs and tinctures with the same goal. I used these drugs during the years when my doctors could not identify my ailment and felt it was predominately mental.

My first reaction was to resist these drugs. I thought they were unnatural and was concerned about becoming dependent on them. I thought taking these drugs made me a weak person. I can trace this belief back to my youth when people felt taking drugs for mental issues was an indicator of mental instability and weakness of character. This "Stone Age" thinking is pure nonsense but it surprisingly has remained in my mind.

When taken with proper medical supervision, the drugs gave me blessed relief. There was no addiction; I was able to stop taking them when the time was right. If at some future time the angst and uncertainty of Crohn's disease becomes intolerable, I would use them again to avoid unnecessary suffering and improve my quality of life. Crohn's disease can be challenging enough without adding uncontrolled mental pain.

Another option for mental suffering is long-term psychological therapy. In my opinion, deep psychoanalysis is not appropriate for episodes of acute mental distress. There is no time for a long discussion to consider past mistakes, the problems of my childhood, or how Crohn's disease has encumbered me. I am hurting and need immediate relief. While my pain may not be physical, my psychological discomfort is intense and can be more distressing than my physical pain. I need either medication or another type of mental therapy to get through these acute episodes.

I could use quick-acting pharmaceuticals to manage my mental pain but instead I have worked to create a variety of quick acting "mental therapies" to help me cope with acute distress. I call this my "emergency mental toolbox."

Emergency Mental Toolbox (EMT)

In times of acute mental distress, I picture a rectangular metal box that is painted glossy white with a big red cross on it. This is a nostalgic image for me, something that I remember from the nurse's office in elementary school. I never saw anyone open it and never observed the contents of this box.

(Who knows—it might have held a package of Hostess Cupcakes or a Hershey's bar. That would have brought a smile and improvement to most any elementary school student in those days.) In my mind, this box had the ability to heal young kids like me and contained some sort of magic. If we were sick or fell down and hurt ourselves, the contents of this emergency kit would heal us.

As a Crohn's patient, I too sometimes have an acute situation and feel psychologically ill, or have fallen down mentally and scraped my mind. During these times, I need a box of "goodies" or tools that I can access quickly for relief. In my mind, I reach for this emergency mental toolbox (or EMT) that contains healing items to relieve my agitated thinking. The ingredients of this EMT provide immediate relief from my anxiety, sadness, anger, or fear. I keep my kit well stocked and update it regularly as new and better ideas come to me.

Shutting off the flame of my discontent

How does this work to help me heal? The tools of my EMT are mental devices that require the use of my creative imagination. *To explain this, I will use the analogy of a skillet and the flame or burner below it.* The skillet represents my mind and the flame underneath represents my feverish thinking process. When I get upset with thoughts of anger, fear, or guilt, this is like turning up the flame too high. If this goes on long enough, the strong flame will eventually make the pan red-hot. This red-hot pan represents my agitated mind as it obsesses and fusses. *In order for me to "cool things down," I need to reduce or turn off this flame underneath my mental skillet.* This means I have to stop obsessing about my challenges; my obsessive thinking is the culprit here. My own mind and inability to cope effectively is making me miserable. Yes, I might have received bad news about my health or had a particularly challenging day. I could have taken this in stride but instead I obsessed about it and created loads of mental agitation. In essence, I turned up the burner that overheated my mind. *The irritating event is only the trigger for my distress; the problem is my poor reaction to it.*

The sequence of how I can become mentally overheated is as follows:

1. First, something bad happens and I react to this in a powerful way and start obsessing about it.

2. This turns up my mental temperature (or the burner flame) and heats the mental skillet, or my mind.

3. As I continue to obsess with thoughts of fear, guilt, or anger, I keep the flame intensely burning and the skillet hot.

In other words, my continued distressful thinking fuels my misery. I need to find various ways to shut off the "mental flame" and thus cool down my mind. I know some gifted people who can do this with their strong willpower; with a few simple thoughts, they can shut off their overactive minds. I am not so lucky and to cool off my obsessive mind, I have to create and then use emergency mental tools from my toolbox. Below are some of the tools that I use:

Using memories to heal

I have a long history of living with Crohn's disease and I can explain this with an extended metaphor. The trail of Crohn's disease has taken me down rough paths and up steep hills (emotional vicissitudes). I have detoured around many a fallen tree (flare), been lost (confused), and found my way by carefully observing the signs along the trail (evaluating my situation). Snakes (unexpected events) have startled me in the grass, and occasionally I have fallen off my horse (given up). However, through persistence and looking for better answers, I found my way back onto the right trail (the path of healing) and have been able to continue the journey. Thus, I have accumulated a valuable storehouse of memories of success in managing Crohn's disease, or life's challenges in general.

When I consider the long history of my experiences with Crohn's, I recognize I have worked through many tough times. I can recall examples of improving after many surgeries, colonoscopies, endoscopies, ERCP's, TPN, hundreds of blood draws, and many emergency room visits. I can visualize how much better I felt after various therapies and observe how my flexibility has increased. There has been pain and mental distress but I dealt with them. I realize that as tough as these experiences are, they do not go on forever. Through my own efforts and the help of my health care team, friends, and family, there is an end to the tunnel of suffering.

These memories of success and working through the many challenges of Crohn's speak to my courage, persistence, stamina, strength, and resilience. I have looked the beast in the eye and been able to move on with my life. Thus, when I am acutely distressed, I recall the memories that prove I have been in a tough situation before and recovered. I can successfully navigate past that scary snake or fallen tree on the trail. It is very calming to recall the history of my successes in dealing with challenging events. These memories restore my confidence and create a powerful antidote to my fear. I am reminded of the old saying, "This too shall pass" as I acknowledge that I have been in situations like this in the past and have survived them. I can do so again with whatever challenges I am confronting today.

Do not make decisions when under stress

I do not make big decisions when upset or dismayed by Crohn's disease. My distressed mind is foggy with whatever emotional upset is active at that moment. I cannot evaluate things carefully and logically or see the big picture. Instead, my world has shrunk to the dimensions of my sickness and distress, and I miss many useful ideas and perspectives.

This caution is standard practice after certain procedures in most clinics and hospitals. For instance, after a colonoscopy or endoscopy, the nursing staff will tell me not to drive or make big decisions until the next day. In fact, I have to sign a paper to this effect. The GI Lab nursing staff at my local hospital will not let me out the door until someone of adult age comes and picks me up. The nursing staff realizes that sedating medication is influencing my reflexes and thinking. I call this "medication jail," and it is strictly enforced.

In the same way, my mental consternation in response to Crohn's disease or another mentally upsetting event influences my mind. Most people will remember the sage advice of parents or friends: take a deep breath and walk away from a situation if you find yourself getting all worked up. Having a serious flare of the disease, needing surgery, or having a bad day at work can place my mind into an emotional funk. I need to put myself in "decision jail" until my short-term state of mental aggravation calms down. I wait for "the sun to come out tomorrow" and in the daylight of feeling better, I am able to use all of my mental faculties and come up with the best evaluation of my situation. I wait until I am mentally calm before making decisions.

Let some time pass

Letting time pass is what I call the "floating technique." I use this in times of extreme distress when I need to step outside of my conscious mind and "float." My mind is in hyperactive mode and cannot seem to slow down. I am mentally frazzled and at my wits end. I need to disconnect my active thinking process for the moment and I do this by letting my mind just float about on whatever topic suits its fancy. This is pulling the plug on my focused thoughts. By doing this, I observe a mass of jumbled and excited thoughts that go whizzing by in my head. It seems like I am burning up excess mental energy. By not focusing or trying to think new thoughts or concentrate, my overheated mental computer eventually slows down. The key point is to float along mentally and let my thoughts come and go without giving them any consideration. In essence, I am "vegging out." No matter what thoughts come up, the idea is to give them no attention and treat them as if they are blowing by in the wind. My aggravated thoughts are the energy behind the storm and if I am able to rest mentally and give little attention to my irritated thoughts, the storm will pass and the winds will dissipate. I might fall asleep or doze off briefly as my mind works to dump the excess overload energy; after some time, my mind settles down and I am able to think clearly again. The storm has passed.

Observing the world

This is a great mental tool to calm me down. When I am mentally in the dumps due to Crohn's, I need to move my attention from inside my head to the outside world around me. When under distress, my own mind becomes a difficult and sometimes nasty place to be. I conjure up all types of ridiculous and scary scenarios. Most of this is pure fantasy but my mind is stuck in this nonsense. When I need a quick way to break out of negative thoughts, here are two options that work well:

1. The first is to shift my attention onto something else that is very engaging. I need to distract myself by finding better things to entertain my mind. This could be a book, a movie, a piece of music, going to the store, or getting together with friends, family, or associates. I do not want to sit in my room in the dark and cogitate on the difficulties going through my mind. When I do that, I energize my nightmarish thoughts and continue to upset myself.

2. The other way to get out of my head involves observing my world and being mindful of its significance. It is very calming to look outside myself. I can remember falling asleep as a child at my grandparents' house. As I started to doze off on the carpet floor, I would hear the soft mumbling of adult voices around me. These voices were very calming and comforting and told me the outside world was still working fine and I could relax and sleep. In a similar way, I can quietly observe people or nearby scenery. I can see order in the world and people going about their days as normal. This process of mindfulness relaxes me and is in sharp contrast to the self-created scary or ghoulish thoughts in my head.

I have used this tool in the hospital when I felt nervous and concerned. I looked at the nursing staff, tuned into the voices around me, and observed the quiet confidence that told me all was well. I have also used this on a bumpy airline flight by observing the flight attendants and most of the passengers taking the bumps and turbulence in stride while they go about resting, reading, watching a movie, or talking. Looking outside of myself helps to pull the plug on my overactive mind. While I might be upset, most people are not and I can tap into their calmness to slow down my distressed mind.

It is not my fault

There are times when I blame myself for a Crohn's disease flare or the fact I have the disease. When something does not go my way, I not only feel whipped by my lack of success but also label myself a failure. I disappoint myself by failing to heal but if I take it a step further and label myself a failure, it is even worse—like a one-two bunch to the gut. This double whammy creates a lot of despair and agitates my mind. This is especially true if I made some progress with Crohn's only to have the problem come back and bite me. It is hard to take this type of disappointment when "the light at the end of the tunnel" turns out to be only a mirage.

This can happen a lot with Crohn's Disease. It ebbs and flows and a flare may surprise me at any time. I need to remember that unpredictability is a regular part of Crohn's disease and to stop blaming myself for something out of my control. It is not the food I ate or something I knowingly did that caused my Crohn's to flare.

So how do I give up my thoughts that I am a failure in managing Crohn's? I remind myself that Crohn's disease has no respect—it comes and goes as it pleases. When Crohn's disease flares, I need to stop beating myself up because this only adds more pain to my moments of tribulation. I am blaming myself for something that is out of my control.

The bumpy course of Crohn's disease is similar to flying on an airplane. I do not like turbulence. I like my seat and surroundings to stay calm and steady so I can move about and relax. But, the reality of flying in an airplane is there are currents of wind outside the plane and these are a normal part of the atmosphere in which the plane flies. As long as there are wind currents and storms in the atmosphere, there will be some bumps along the way. In the same way, as long as there is Crohn's disease, there will be bumps along the way. There is not a whole lot I can do other than follow the advice of professionals and take care of myself. My health care professionals are like the pilots of the planes who try to keep the ride smooth, but unexpected turbulence is normal. In the same way I do not blame the pilot for the wind currents or turbulence, I do not blame my physicians for flares. Giving myself grief for something that is both normal for this type of disease and beyond my control is ridiculous. As I come to accept Crohn's disease for what it is and how it behaves, I help reduce my agitation.

My creative mind can produce monsters

When I think about all of my problems with Crohn's disease over the years, the problems that I imagine in my head are worse than what actually happens. This is even true with surgery and recovery. My imaginings about the side effects to drugs, the pain from surgery, the length of my flare, or the loss of my hope and livelihood are always overblown compared to reality. Even some of the toughest times have not been as bad as I had imagined. By reminding myself of my tendency to catastrophize, I can help cool my irritated mind.

Having dealt with this for decades, I have learned the source of my catastrophic thoughts is not my doctors, family, or friends. It is a young and immature part of me that I have named the "boy who cried wolf"; my "department of fear"; or my 'immature self." This immature part of me likes to foretell all my future miseries. It tells me that my current episode of Crohn's is going to mushroom into a disaster even though this frequently never happens. Catastrophic thinking is using my creative imagination in a destructive way. I can use my imagination and memories to heal, but I can also use it to harm and create more mental pain. I have learned to quietly and firmly remind myself that catastrophic thoughts are harmful to my health and to give them no mind. I have created new tools including a multistep program to manage my "department of fear" or "immature self" and I write about this in later chapters.

Using my mind/body connection

If I can create more comfort in my body, my mind will relax and calm down. Taking a warm shower/bath or a massage are two such examples. For me, the feel of the warm water on my skin is relaxing and leaves me feeling mentally clean and refreshed even if I am distressed. I can say the same for massage: I can feel the tenderness and attention in the masseuse's hands. This translates into a sense of personal comfort and some relief from my overactive mind.

Walking is another favorite tool of mine. It seems to help with moving my digestion along and is refreshing to my mind. By walking outside, there are many things to observe; looking outwardly helps to distract my mind from any lingering nasty thoughts. Because my mind is distracted, my mental temperature of agitation drops and life is brighter. I walk two or three miles each day—have done so for decades—and it is a quick and easy way to deal with mental distress. I am frequently "on the road again" as I walk through various neighborhoods come rain or shine. I have met all of the neighborhood dogs, observed which neighbor is moving out or who has moved in, observed who bought a new car, noticed houses newly painted or tented for termites, and admired new landscaping. Walking is my favorite physical tool for mental distress and it comes with many side benefits, such as excellent blood pressure and stamina.

Mental shower

A "mental shower" is a tool of my creative imagination. I use this tool in the shower but it could be performed anywhere. I have already mentioned that a good warm shower tends to clear my head. Adding in a mental shower gives me even better results to cleanse my overactive mind. The idea is that just as I accumulate dirt throughout the day, I also accumulate the mental dirt of anger, guilt, or fear. This accumulated mental dirt is irritating and I must wash it away. I use the following mental exercise to remove it.

As I feel the warm relaxing water on my body, I observe the background noise of my own thoughts. Are my thoughts agitated, angry, and upset? Are they fearful, sad, or full of guilt? There is no attempt to analyze any of these thoughts; I just make note of them. After a few moments, I tell any thoughts of anger, fear, or guilt that I am letting them go. I do this kindly, gently, and with love, not forcefully. I smile internally and then ask my upsetting thoughts to leave. They simply exit my body and the warm water washes them away. After making this request, I have a clear mental image of my nasty thoughts and irritation washing down the drain along with the soap and dirt from my body. I even look at the drain below and mentally wave goodbye as they disappear.

This whole exercise might sound very strange for those who do not work with visualizations, but it works well for me. My chatter of overactive consternating thoughts is like dirt in my carpet or the background noise of loud traffic along a freeway. There is no need for me to try to analyze this dirt or talk over this type of noise—instead, I just wash it away. When I sweep the floor, I do not evaluate the dirt, determine where it came from, or analyze what it means. I consider it to be a part of daily living and sweep it away. I can use this mental exercise while sitting in a chair or taking a walk but I enjoy using this thought process in a shower because I can clean both my mental and physical self at the same time. The more I practice this technique, the better it works.

Quick prayer

I am not an expert on prayer, but it is part of my life. I do not have training in religious prayer or its use in a church so I use a simple prayer that is straightforward. For me it always starts with making sure I have done all that I can to remedy a situation. My prayer then goes something like this: "(God, Spirit, and Lord) I am doing all that I can and need your help. I need your help with my acute physical pain/mental distress/anger/fear/sadness/frustration. I know you are the source of all strength, courage, stamina, and health in my life and as I ask for your blessings now, I am grateful and thankful for this answered prayer."

This type of urgent prayer is useful and it brings me relief to the challenges of the moment. My clear expectation is this prayer will work and be answered. I am firm in my conviction and deeply appreciate this support. My prayer is heartfelt and I commit myself to using the added health I receive to be useful in my activities.

While I use these tools for acute situations, they can also work when my issues are not as pronounced. For example, there are days that I might be mildly irritable or fearful: I feel out of sorts and cranky, but cannot attribute it to anything. I have run down my tank of optimism and goodwill and it needs to recharge. I help myself by floating, using the mental shower, letting some time pass, and using my mind/body connection through walking. All of these tend to help clear away my cobwebs and defuse some of my irritation.

My proven mental EMT and the tools contained within are an important part of how I manage my Crohn's disease for urgent problems and crises. These tools are not a permanent treatment for Crohn's, but can serve as band-aids to get me through the day. I still have more involved work to do with my mind, emotions and spirit. Because I have used these tools in my EMT with regularity, they have become a common part of my thinking process and I also use them when I experience meltdowns not associated with Crohn's disease.

When I first started developing the tools, I had to go through them slowly to retrain my mind to think differently. As my mind learned of their power and appreciated their effectiveness, these mental tasks were easier to perform. When I am severely flustered, it may take longer to obtain good results, but these tools eventually work to turn off the burner of irritated thoughts and calm my internal temperature of inflammation. These quick-acting mental tools are integral when seeking rapid relief from my distress with Crohn's disease. Undoubtedly, there are additional tools I have yet to discover, but these I have described have been thoroughly tested and found to be extremely useful.

Chapter 8 — The Bully of Crohn's Disease

I am not a psychologist, nor am I steeped in intimate knowledge of the human psyche, but there are significant negative emotions that affect my well-being. What does this have to do with Crohn's disease? Living with Crohn's tends to bring out my destructive emotions. It is easy to understand why as I look at how Crohn's behaves.

How Crohn's would behave if it were an actual person

What follows is a description of how Crohn's would behave if it came alive as a walking and talking person. I'll name him Mr. Crohn's. First of all, he always drops in unannounced. He comes and goes as he pleases and might show up after a hard day at work, at my daughter's wedding, on my anniversary or my birthday. You would think that he would be kind enough to at least call, send a telegram, or text me that he is on his way. However, he just comes barging in at the most inopportune time. This behavior is irritating and frustrating which increases my mental inflammation.

Mr. Crohn's has this obnoxious habit of punching me in the stomach. I might be enjoying a nice movie and then bam, a punch to the gut. Alternatively, I might be at work trying to finish a report or visiting at home with friends and then find myself unable to sit comfortably in a chair because of pain.

Mr. Crohn's does not care how well my life is going or what other issues I am managing. If I have a bad cold, hurt my arm, or have a toothache, he continues to demand my attention like a whiny child. He behaves the same way when I have a tight deadline at work or an issue with a sick child. He is not willing to respond to my needs, give me a break, or let me live a normal life.

He gives me a chronic case of indigestion and pain. Eating with him is frightening as I am unsure how he will react to my next meal. Some food that seemed agreeable in the past might create waves of nausea or a quick run to the bathroom. This act of terror can destroy a pleasant evening at a restaurant with friends.

He is famous for conjuring up new areas of discomfort. When previously I have never experienced a pain in my left side, he decides that I should see how that feels and I get a new pain in my left side. On the other hand, he might scare me by turning my toilet bowl water blood-red. He is devious as well when he decides to disappear for a long stretch of time. He will become a distant memory but then when I least expect it, BAM! He storms through the door and calls out for me to drop everything, for he is back!

To sum it up, Mr. Crohn's is insensitive, obnoxious, narcissistic, self-absorbed, and a real bully who picks at people indiscriminately.

A personified acquaintance like Mr. Crohn's would be a nightmare to live with, and yet I—along with other tens of thousands of other Crohn's patients—do so each day. This is my permanent lifelong reality. If I am going to live with a terrorist bully like Mr. Crohn's, I must find effective ways to manage myself physically, mentally and emotionally to reduce his ability to create serious havoc. This requires an EMT kit for emergencies and many other self-management tools and ideas.

It is easy to be resentful of Crohn's disease. It seems natural to want to lash out in anger at my condition, but surprisingly this makes it worse. If I treat the illness in myself as a hostile presence, I will regard it as a permanent enemy and be at constant war with this part of me. I will bond with it on the wavelength of resentment. This action of detesting a part of myself undermines healing at all levels. Self-healing (as described in this chapter and elsewhere in this book) requires tolerance, patience, understanding, and nurturing love—not anger and rejection. I cannot fight Crohn's disease directly because I only end up fighting myself. Instead, I must learn to reform my responses, attitudes and beliefs associated with it and build health.

Mind/body connection

Finding better ways to manage my mental and emotional self has significantly helped my symptoms and well-being. Many people have heard of a mind and body connection, as I wrote about in Chapter 7. Whenever I increase my burner flame and experience anger, guilt, or fear, I feel it immediately in my gut or solar plexus. This pattern repeats itself in me like clockwork.

For example, let's say something happens in my life such as

having a disagreement with a friend or a client feeling my services were unsatisfactory. Perhaps I burnt dinner or was not mentally prepared to handle another endoscopy. I respond to these events with my emotional experiences of anger or fear. As I experience these emotions, I can feel the "tightening" of my solar plexus area: a sharp burning sensation in my gut accompanied by painful spasms in my belly. I experience physical along with emotional and mental pain when I become angry or fearful. My upset gut, with observable inflammation, cannot handle significant emotional and mental upset—it is like pouring salt on an open wound. This is a great motivator for me to do everything I can to manage it.

I have pondered if my years of chronic anger and fear could have either triggered the beginning of Crohn's disease or served as a catalyst for a recurrence or flare. I have never seen such a study and cannot imagine how to design one. I have read anecdotal experiences and my own reality indicates excessive fatigue or stress exacerbates Crohn's disease. My firsthand experience tells me there is a strong association between stress and increased symptoms. Maybe chronic irritation of my gut due to anger, fear, or guilt influences my normal immune response and makes things worse. Once again, there is no way to prove this. However, I know my mental distress exacerbates my symptoms and this is a good enough reason for me to do something about it to promote health and comfort.

Mental and emotional baggage

In order to heal my anger, guilt, fear, or even resentment, pessimism, or disgust, I must first acknowledge I have a problem. I find this difficult. I do not always see the type of person I really am. I rarely admit to being hostile, moody, irritable, outright nasty, or fearful. I see myself in a positive light and it is hard to look in the mirror and see otherwise. I have never met anyone who routinely openly confesses to being an obnoxious, fearful, or angry person. While they might admit to occasional outbursts of irritation, they genuinely feel they are regular people who are pleasant to be around. Alternatively, if they are upset, they think they have good reasons to feel this way. I, too, can justify my own anger or fear because of some outward event and not my own issue of a lack of self-control.

Seeing my irritations and mental issues as damaging to my welfare and the welfare of others requires me to look beyond my outward demeanor and deeper into myself, versus denying my negativity or rationalizing it with the easy excuse that, even if I am angry and anxious, this is a "normal" response and completely natural. I must learn to see there are alternative ways to behave instead of getting upset.

I must also see past my idea that I will always be at least mildly irritable, fearful, or guilt-ridden. I learned to accept that my baseline of unhealthy emotions was perfectly "normal" as long as they were not significant enough to create major problems. Nobody told me that I could do better and actually change my emotional personality to a new baseline. Even as I began my mental and emotional work with Crohn's disease and tried to eliminate my larger mood swings that were clearly destructive, I did not know that I could actually change my baseline of emotional and mental health. However, after working with my overall program for managing Crohn's disease, I recognized that my background or baseline levels of emotional angst and good emotions have changed for the better. This was an unexpected bonus of all my work and significantly improved my well-being and joy.

In order to see how I really behave, I ask myself a few simple questions:

- Do I constantly fret about my health, job, and/or relationships?

- Is my daily mood normally light and easy or is it crabby?

- Do I feel overwhelmed on a regular basis?

- Do I think and worry about my next Crohn's flare even when things are going well?

- Am I regularly dismayed at the humiliation and loss of control that Crohn's brings into my life?

- Do I have recurring irritating issues with my boss, family members, and friends?

- When I take time off on weekends or vacations, do I have a good time or end up fussing, and fretting?

- Do I get upset as I think about how others take advantage of and do not respect me?

- Do I tend to put people off or see people as incompetent or inferior?

- Am I often critical or angry with myself?

- Do the little problems of life tend to bug me?

- Am I always putting myself down and feeling bad

about my performance?

- Do I spend time reliving old wounds and recreating my pain?

The answers to these types of questions tells me if I have a problem with mental and emotional control and am not as calm, joyful, and self-controlled as I hoped. I find I might also harbor a lot of bottled-up emotions and mental pain. Some people like me may exhibit outward self-control (remain calm and polite in demeanor) but in fact be stuffing themselves full of anger, guilt and fear. *I have learned my self-loathing and self-disgust is just as toxic as my loathing and disgust of others or life events and I must moderate these negative emotions if I want to heal.* While pretending to handle life with ease can be useful socially, it does not negate the damage done by the bottled-up internal turmoil. This just buries the stress deeper in my body, making everything worse, and can lead to other psychological pathologies like passive-aggressive behavior, depression, or chronic anxiety. There are better choices (to be described later) that truly bring healing.

My work on mental and emotional health is not a passive process or a "quick fix." For many years, my response to stressful events was avoidance, denial, or practicing a passive form of meditation. If things got tough, it was easy to go somewhere and relax, do yoga, take a nap, exercise, ignore it or meditate. While these exercises seemed to help briefly, they did not directly address my mental and emotional issues; thus, these issues came back after a brief respite.

Working with my mental and emotional state is not easy. I have many habits that are ingrained in me and are resistant to change.

They are like bodyguards that protect my outdated behavior and responses while making it difficult to improve my character and develop better self-control. I need first-class tools and strong motivation to do this work. Surprisingly, the pain of Crohn's disease is a strong motivator to do this heavy lifting. After trying medications, diet and exercise to get rid of the plague of Crohn's and failing, my only remaining opportunity for better health and personal growth was through cleaning up my unhealthy emotional and mental attitudes and beliefs.

Healing my mental and emotional wounds can take time but I can do something each day to help the process. The process of helping my body heal from a physical wound can teach me a lot about how to heal my mental and emotional wounds.

<u>When I am physically wounded, I need to:</u>

1. Give my body rest and eat well.

2. Take pain medication.

3. Do not obsess and fuss about my physical wound but instead realize that it will take time to heal.

4. Apply healing liniments as needed.

5. Do not pick at or rub the wound but instead leave it alone or protect it.

6. As I become stronger, I can carefully learn to work with this wounded part of my body and develop a more active routine.

Thus, when I am wounded psychologically, I need to:

1. Give my mind rest, eat well, and avoid making big decisions.

2. Take psychological medications like antidepressants or sleeping aids, if needed.

3. Do not allow myself to fuss and fret about how wounded I am but instead allow time to pass so I can heal.

4. Wash and apply salve to my mental wound by flushing away my negative responses and giving myself nurturing thoughts and ideas.

5. Do not pick at my wound by repeatedly reliving the hurt. I need to leave it alone for now.

6. As I become stronger, I can carefully approach my psychological wound and impart wisdom and nourishing love as needed. This internal psychological dialogue is part of a 7-step process I outline in later chapters.

I have a number of key emotional responses that give me a significant challenge. I would like to identify these emotions, along with the different mental tools I use to manage them. My motivation is to reduce my psychological irritation that is also influencing my experiences of Crohn's disease in my body. *While there are many emotional responses to consider, the big three that influence me are anger, fear, and guilt and their corresponding cousins, irritation, anxiety and shame.*

My goal in working with anger, fear, and guilt is to moderate them, bring them under better control, and thereby minimize their ability to create havoc in my life. By doing so, I can reduce my mental and physical irritation and better manage the various trials and tribulations of Crohn's disease.

Chapter 9 — Relief from Intimidating Fear

Fear—and its cousin, anxiety—are my most significant negative emotional experiences and they mercilessly aggravate my gut. The origin of my fear reaction is uncertain but as I wrote in Chapter 7, "the boy who cried wolf" is likely a significant source of my immature protective mechanism that creates a lot of grief for me. When I developed much of this as a young child, I had no idea there were other ways to deal with anxious moments. In the past, I listened to all the "boy who cried wolf" had to say as he foretold my future miseries. He would tell me that my current episode of Crohn's or other life challenges were going to mushroom into disasters. Even though his frightening premonitions were usually wrong, I believed them.

I have sometimes wondered where the voice of "the boy who cried wolf" comes from. What caused my mind to come up with these disaster scenarios? This must have been a protective device I created as a young child. This voice of caution was there to warn me of some possible dangerous situations. As an adult, I can see the bigger picture and the patterns of recurrences, and thus make sense of it all; this was not possible as a child.

Growing up, my response to potential danger was very basic and dominated by fear, anger, and guilt. This was my full repertoire of ways to fight the danger. *My fear response was for me to run away, my anger response was for me to fight back and my guilt response was that it was my fault.* When I look at my issues today, I see these basic responses are outdated and no longer necessary. Furthermore, these behaviors have not only outlived their usefulness, they are now a determent and can actually fan the flames of my overheated obsessive mind.

Today, the "boy who cried wolf" is still a part of my life. He has not fully gone away; occasionally, in a moment of acute distress, he shows up yet again with his cries of disaster. I can hear his angry or fearful or guilt-ridden voice warning me that things are going to get worse or a calamity is about to happen. However, with the adult part of me, I can now take the boy aside and let him know that while I appreciate his concern, his efforts are no longer necessary. The adult part of me will take over and make sure we are safe and my life is in good order, as it relates to Crohn's disease and life's issues. I suggest to this little boy that he can now use his energies for other things besides warning me. I tell him to do what the youthful part of me is designed to do: use his many great attributes such as creativity, enthusiasm, playfulness, and joy to help me grow in life, rather than crippling me with fear about catastrophic threats. *These are important parts of me I can put to good use.*

In psychological terms, I do not know what this "boy" is or how he relates to my psyche; this kind of information is not important to me. What I do know is that this "little boy" is a permanent part of my psychological makeup, and I will try to find a useful role for him. Because he is part of me, I treat him with respect. It would be easy for me to berate this part of myself for its immaturity and inability to see things more clearly. However—particularly as a Crohn's patient—yelling at myself will only generate more internal turmoil and aggravation, increasing my mental agitation. Thus, I instead choose to counsel and work with these immature parts of my makeup.

In essence, I am having an internal dialogue with several different but equally important parts of myself: the adult and childlike elements. Through this dialogue, I help them to work together to create a positive mental environment that serves me well as I deal with Crohn's disease and other life challenges. Through these dialogues, I have learned how to handle cries of "Danger! Danger!" or "Disaster ahead!" from the childlike part of my mind. I no longer heed his calls, but I am able to speak to this "little boy who called wolf." I ask him to stop making me angry or scared and instead express creativity and enthusiasm about something constructive. By doing so, I further cool down my overly distressed mind and stop expecting disaster at every turn.

Fear is not something I either can or wish to eliminate from my life. It can function well as a healthy caution, calling attention to potentially dangerous situations. However, in its extreme or chronic form, it is excessive, destructive, and irritates my mind and bowels. Along with life's normal challenges, Crohn's disease has taken me down this road of excessive fear as I have dealt with pain, procedures, bowel issues, and surgeries. It is time for me to take control and reduce the impact of this self-induced mental irritation.

Managing fear requires me to set the scene and create a good working environment between my adult and childish components. I must remain focused, so I cannot successfully have this type of dialogue as I drive my car, watch TV, or am otherwise preoccupied. The following outline is how I set up and converse with my childlike self who controls my excessive fear.

In preparation for this internal dialogue, I want to avoid the mistake of considering whatever is bad, irritating, or unpleasant as an "enemy." If I do so, I will treat it as such and hate it, reject it, or try to punish or destroy it. In this instance, my immature fear is a part of me and if I wage war on it through hateful or punishing techniques, I just add to my misery—almost like hitting my own hand with a hammer in response to my mistakes. I must manage this immature part of myself in a similar way that I would teach and discipline a small child. Harsh methods would only alienate a child and increase fear, anger, and guilt. Therefore, I use a kind, compassionate tone in the following seven steps of my dialogue with my childlike self.

1. Being gentle and nurturing

I need to be gentle and nurturing when working with the immature elements within myself. My fear communicates in very basic terms; thus, when I speak to this part of me, I need to approach it as I would a very young child and talk to it with calmness. I need to show respect, understanding, and eliminate all self-effacing, derogatory, and nasty comments. Using terms like stupid, dumb, idiot, lazy, or inept towards this part of me will shut down all ability to communicate or make contact. Through this gentle approach, I can develop a relationship of trust as I use the adult part of me to take over the responsibility of managing challenging life events like Crohn's disease.

When I first work on an issue and my wound is fresh and intense, this might be all I can accomplish in my first dialogue with my immature self. It reminds me of what my grandmother would do if I had just fallen down and skinned my knee or failed at something. My dismay would be overwhelming and she would be there to comfort me while I calmed down. My grandmother would rock me in a chair as I lay on her lap. They were no words spoken, but I experienced her nurturing touch and acceptance that was like a healing balm for my troubled mind. It is what I needed. Only after I had calmed down would she start to speak and help me process my hurt and pain. This is exactly what I do for myself as I lay my wounded self on my "mental lap" and rock it while pouring forth nourishing and caring energies from my adult self.

2. Expressing thanks

I need to express thanks to my childlike self. He has done his best to keep me safe in the only way he knew how. By expressing thanks, I acknowledge that he is a worthy contributor to my psyche. *This helps my childlike self build confidence and recognize the value he has created in my life over many decades.* He was motivated to protect me from further failure, embarrassment, loss, humiliation, or possible calamity. However, just being thankful to him is not the end of my work because I still must make the appropriate changes to this part of me. Otherwise, I will only have excused my fear without correcting it. I need to educate my childlike self to adopt a more intelligent version of protecting me that incorporates additional wisdom and skills. To be concerned about threats to my well-being is good, but I must express these concerns in a more effective and healthy way.

3. Asking for help

I need to ask my childlike self to help me reduce my fearful response. This part of me has been and still is the major driver of my excessively fearful reactions and I need his involvement to bring my fear under control. I cannot have him throwing a tantrum and disrupting my need to make changes. By asking for his help, I am also embracing him as an important part of my life. *I am addressing my childlike self with respect and not as an inferior or flawed part of my makeup. However, I am not asking for this help as an equal. This relationship is more like a parent and child, with the parent possessing greater wisdom, compassion, and authority. Ultimately, my childlike elements need to understand and embrace adult rules and strategies as the new standard for healthy living.* Expressing respect for the intelligence and value of the childlike components of me while asking for help is significant in building a bridge of communication—but I must be clear that the adult me is in charge.

4. Imparting perspective (or an intelligent view), wisdom (or knowledge and skill), and love (gratitude, nurturing, kindness, patience etc.)

This is the counseling part of my conversation with my childlike self. It is what my grandmother or close relatives used to do when they imparted wisdom and helped me gain perspective on an upsetting situation. I explain to my immature self that times have changed and he now has help from the more mature part of me. He no longer has to bear the full burden of keeping us safe with his strong sense of fear. Instead, he can relax and know that a mature part of us is on the job handling life's challenging issues. I talk with him about the situation and offer adult perspective and insights. I do not make this overly complex, but give enough information to allow my fearful part to release control over the situation. *In essence, I am offering to establish a partnership with my fearful self in which I am bringing my superior mental and emotional abilities to help. I am imparting wisdom based upon experience and maturity while creating a partnership and maintaining control of the situation.*

This is important because the dark side of my personality, when hurt, often behaves like a small child that goes off and hides in the corner for his own protection. That is, this type of dialogue could lead to hurt feelings on the part of my childlike self. It is not unlike constructive criticism I get at work. While this is useful and necessary and I may welcome it, sometimes part of me feels hurt. I might sulk off into my office, becoming isolated and withdrawn. Psychologically, this isolation of my childlike self separates him from my best qualities of intelligence, patience, tolerance, forgiveness, courage—the very qualities that I need for healing. By offering a partnership with my childlike self, I am offering him respect and bringing him into a greater light of health and wisdom. This is an essential step to healing.

I have learned that as I impart my wisdom, perspective, and love to this immature part of me, smaller aggravations melt away: the specifics of what happened, who "did it" to me, why I have to deal with this, or where this hurt originated no longer seem important. While it might be intellectually interesting to work through such things, frequently it does not matter. In fact, the origins of many of my bad habits are hard to trace and have become distorted over time. In addition, there are no good answers to why I am bullied by Crohn's disease; I just am. Even if the situation has nothing to do with Crohn's—for example, if I have a difficult time with my manager at work or an argument with my family—sorting through all of the details, establishing blame, and trying to prosecute the guilty party does not usually result in healing. It usually leads to more frustration and reliving the whole painful experience all over again. With few exceptions, most of my healing comes through self-nurturing and perspective.

As my adult self takes over the responsibility of managing a wound or hurt, my nurturing helps to heal the wound through patience and loving attention. I can also add in mature ideas and thoughts that further allow me to ameliorate my fearful and aggravated response. Some of these perspectives include:

- I am a work in progress but filled with latent strengths, wisdom, creativity, and dignity.

- I have many gifts and good possibilities.

- I can overcome my character flaws and live my life more gracefully.

- I can view my strengths of character and use them in difficult situations

- I might have made some errors but I can learn from them, improve my skills, and do better next time…all is not lost.

- I need to determine if I might be too sensitive, timid, cynical, self-absorbed, or hostile

- Sometimes I need to put myself in another person's shoes, to see things from their side, and use that perspective to mute my excessive emotionalism.

- I need to be cautious that some of my excessive reactions are to blame others for my own issues because I think I am overly special and deserving of exceptional treatment and not subject to the rules that others must follow.

5. Asking about his needs

I ask my immature self what else I can do for him.

- Am I ignoring any of his basic needs?

- Are there other issues I have failed to address or uncover?

- If so, what are they?

The purpose behind these questions is to identify any unknown or unmet internal wishes. This is what we do as good parents at home or good supervisors at work. We regularly ask our children or employees what we can do to help them in order to uncover any unmet needs before things get out of hand. It is common to have unmet needs, which is why it is critical to actively look for them. It has taken me decades to realize that I have a childlike part of me that is struggling and it makes sense there are various issues that I have not yet uncovered. It is important that as I ask these questions, I listen and when an answer comes, I take action. Only in this way do I build confidence in the childlike part of myself that he can trust me to be there with better ideas and useful answers.

I have also noticed that a motivating force that recreates fear is often some irrational or silly problem that has long since vanished. For example, I can remember my mother taking me to the doctor when I was very young and each time she would say it was "not a big deal." However, with most visits I would get poked and prodded and usually end up with either a blood draw or a shot. Thus, I began to fear going to the doctor as a painful process and associate the smell of the doctor's office with that pain. My small mind could see no value or healing from going to a doctor, only pain and discomfort. Even as an adult, the faint smell of the doctor's office set off this uncomfortable reaction, but I now understand why and have moved to correct it. The same is true with my responses to certain types of people if I continue to use outdated and immature methods of communication.

I have found my childish elements do not behave rationally. This can lead to monsters in my mind but through patiently and quietly asking for input on any needs, even the "childish" ones, I can recognize that the monsters never existed and were just a phantom of my imagination and fears. My childlike self often acts as if he does not truly understand that I have grown up and become a mature, resourceful adult. As an adult speaking to the child, I have to convey this message in very clear, firm, and compassionate terms. I understand that this part of me has been quite isolated from the rest of me and as such did not feel supported—he never knew that we grew up and outgrew some of these silly fears.

6. *This is a team effort*

I need my childlike self to be on my team and to work with me. His childishness remains within me and I must work on it, but this childlike part of me also brings forth great qualities that are important parts of my character. I send my childish elements the message that collectively as a team we can work together to make our life what we want. While childlike parts of me have value, I must use careful surgery to separate them from the childish qualities that are unhealthy. The immature parts of me may perceive value in stubbornness, anger, fear, or guilt; therefore, I must use my mature, adult mind to manage these negative emotions.

7. *A lifelong commitment*

I must let my childlike self know that I will check in frequently to assess his needs. When I start this dialogue, I convey that this is not a one-time conversation and the plan is to check in with this childlike part of me on a regular basis. I have learned that as a supervisor, a good father, and a spouse, my relationships require regular attention. *I take a few minutes at the end of each day to create confidence in my childlike self that I am on the job and taking care of any challenging issues that could overwhelm him.* Moreover, if I notice my childlike self communicating through his blast of acute fear, anger, or guilt, I will stop and take the time to listen and respond.

Some readers might find this exercise a little strange; you might think the idea of a childlike element in yourself is silly or ridiculous, or that this process is a waste of time and will not work for you. However, this program has worked wonders for me in addressing my significant damaging issues of fear, guilt, and anger. The process started when I first asked myself: do I have chronic issues with guilt, anger, or fear? The answer was yes and I recognized I had work to do. With this 7-step program, I can connect with the childlike part of me, listen to his needs, and let him know he is an important part of my life even though his role of protector and use of childish tools is over. I have better adult ideas and solutions to handle difficult challenges. As my mature self takes charge, I have found my fearful (or angry, or guilty) reactions are on the decline. I cannot fully explain the science or psychology behind how it all works, but it does.

This is not the end of my efforts to manage excessive fear, anger or guilt. In this chapter, I discussed ways to begin healing the reactionary and fearful childish elements of myself. I also have the tools in my EMT, as discussed in Chapter 7, to catch and quell those acute flare-ups of fear, anger or guilt. In addition, later in this book I will go into my work of healing distorted beliefs and thoughts; bringing in significant transformative qualities of gratitude, forgiveness, and joy; and working with spiritual forces. All of these strategies work together to quell my issues with fear, anger and guilt. However, as discussed in this chapter, making an internal connection with the frightful, angry, or guilt-ridden part of me is a significant starting point on the path of healing and developing a more mature character.

Chapter 10 — Cooling Inflammatory Anger

Anger and irritation are the second-most prevalent emotional experiences for me to manage. My anger is not explosive, but rather manifests as a slow irritating burn. When things do not go smoothly, I get irritated and this can encompass my work, my home life, and Crohn's disease. Over time, this seething anger heats up my mind, then my body, and is something I cannot tolerate as a Crohn's patient.

Nobody likes being around angry, irritated people. My excessive anger is a childish part of my personality, just like excessive fear. My childlike self is using anger to both protect me and to fight for what it wants (whether deserved or not.) This angry part of myself lashes out to get his way and can be a true bully at times. His actions are not rational but are a very basic protective confrontational mechanism. He attacks not only my perceived physical dangers of potential violence or loss of home or family, but my psychological dangers of humiliation, loss of opportunity, failure, and regret. Other situations that might elicit anger include:

- not being able to do things perfectly

- thinking others are ripping me off

- being frustrated that I cannot accomplish my projects at work

- experiencing money problems

- having an argument with a family member

- suffering from a Crohn's flare

- thinking nobody understands the pain I am experiencing

- dwelling on the unfairness of having Crohn's

One can argue that all of these issues are valid and it would be acceptable to be angry or irritated by them. I find that while it might seem sensible to be angry in these situations, this anger does not help me with my Crohn's disease or life in general. Being angry has never helped me be a better person or solve my greatest problems. Getting all worked up does not make my gut feel lighter. It does not bring more peace to my mind. On the contrary, being angry increases the "burner flame" of my irritation and hurts my ability to be a better parent, father, boss, friend, and mentor.

On the plus side, anger can give me added strength if I need it to protect myself in a life-threatening situation, but this is extremely rare. Instead, using my anger excessively in mundane situations has toxic effects that further aggravate my experience of Crohn's disease and wreak havoc with my relationships.

Some might argue that anger is justified and if I do not express it, I am harming myself by denying my feelings. I would respond to this concern by clarifying that I never deny my own thoughts or feelings. Instead, I try to listen to their messages and then choose how to respond. My departments of fear, anger, or guilt call my attention to issues that I need to work on. While their responses of anger, fear, and guilt are childish, there might be valid issues that my adult mind needs to manage. I can choose to be angry or not with an employee, my daughters, my wife, or Crohn's disease. As a Crohn's patient, I have learned to make it a top priority to keep down my flame of irritation and anger, both to benefit me and my other relationships. Feeling entitled to be angry is a stiff price to pay because if I harbor and spew out anger, it tears me up inside and hurts those around me.

This does not mean I become a victim, have a pity party, and do nothing. When I notice a rising irritation over an event, this is a time I take action to correct or relieve the issue. I look for better answers and concrete solutions. I might feel a bit of testiness and mild irritation as I work through my problems, but I remind myself that I cannot afford to have my irritations escalate or become overwhelming and malevolent. *I can still stand up for myself and work to resolve issues, but I do so in a calm and thoughtful manner, without anger. This is not only supportive to my health, it also gives me better results.* Issues are resolved more efficiently and permanently when I calm down and use better skills of communication.

As I explained in the previous chapter about dealing with fear, I work to resolve anger by opening a dialogue with my childlike self. I take some time every day to express loving respect, thoughtfulness, helpfulness, commitment, and thankfulness to this childlike, important part of me. If I am experiencing anger, I patiently use the mature part of myself to speak with my angry part via the 7-step program described before. As with fear, this is an internal dialogue, it takes time, and I must do it regularly. I cannot take a hiatus from this work, just as I cannot take a hiatus from working on my other life relationships. It is a lifelong commitment to keep my anger and irritation under better control.

I want to share one other program I tried in the distant past to manage my anger. This was a popular method of "letting it all out" by blasting my anger towards whomever I felt deserved it, beating up a pillow, or yelling at the universe. This ultimate self-indulgent program advised that screaming my anger towards anyone I felt deserved it was the best form of treatment. By doing this, I would clear away all of my pent-up, angry baggage. The solution to all of my issues was to tear into the person or situation that offended me with a full blast of anger. They needed to hear how I really felt and feel my wrath. I thought that if I did this, I would feel fantastic. In the same way, I pointed my anger at my own body and yelled expletives at my inflamed bowels, and cursed my body for all the problems it has caused. I was optimistic that spewing out all of my anger would bring blessed relief to my internal pain and would give me new strength and confidence.

If this had helped me to feel better and heal, I might still be doing it. *However, this "letting it all out" tool was a total disaster for me. While I did experience some short-term relief because of the exhilaration of appearing to defeat my enemies, I was left exhausted.* I also alienated others around me and did not reduce the pain of my Crohn's disease. The long-term results were lousy and this technique did not improve any of my relationships. It just made things worse.

It is important to mention the necessity of being patient with this type of work, be it for anger, fear, or guilt. It is possible that as you do this work, you will experience immediate relief from excessive emotions. However, it is more likely that this process will take time, as it has for me. I have wondered why I cannot quickly fix my destructive emotions. I am an adult now, so I should be able to take care of this, right? Why am I not able to have a good adult-to-child conversation with my childlike self and solve the problem once and for all? The key word here is "childlike." I know by experience that when my children were young, they did not always hear me or truly understand what I was saying to them. Children do not have the sophisticated mental and emotional tools or self-control to evaluate various situations, put them in perspective, and make the necessary adjustments. Alternatively, if they do respond right away, they frequently forget about it soon after. For my childish self, the learning process requires lots of patience, repetition, and time.

Furthermore, it is important to remember that my immature self has acted unchecked for decades. This also contributes to the slow process of doing this type of work. After so many years, my strong negative habits are now automatic, so I have to take my brain off autopilot, install new mental software, reboot my emotional programs, and then work to debug them. This process can be challenging and takes time, but the net effect is a much better psychological operating program that does not frequently crash and burn.

My program of self-improvement requires a proactive approach of developing specific strengths, adopting new skills, and giving suitable praise and encouragement. As my own coach and cheerleader, I acknowledge my progress. I also accept my responsibility for this process and commit to make the necessary reforms and amendments as necessary.

One important lesson I have learned is that my outward expressions of anger, fear or guilt must match my internal experiences. This means I cannot "hide" my thoughts of anger, fear, or guilt. If I appear outwardly calm and yet am full of angst on the inside, I have a big problem. When my inside world and outside world are in conflict, I set myself up for a lot of internal turmoil, hurt, and suffering. I can change my outward behavior, but in order to create real health I must also change my inward emotional experiences so all parts of my self are in sync.

Medication and psychotherapy are reasonable tools to employ if needed. For me, my approach thus far has been to rework my mental software on my own. This has been an effective solution. However, others might benefit from additional tools as well. Medication can reduce or blunt the experience of anger, fear, and guilt, but I am reluctant to depend on medication because it will do nothing to modify my belief system, standards, or my sense of identity—the elements that keep recreating anger, fear, and guilt. Psychotherapy with a doctor or counselor is another option. In fact, what I have described via my 7-step program is a simple, self-directed psychotherapy that I do on my own.

Can I use a similar methodology as described for anger or fear to work with other excessive negative emotions like sadness, grief, or cynicism? Can I address them in the same manner? I have done limited work on my other "immature qualities" such as these and the tools I presented here were useful. As can be seen with the two examples of fear and anger, I need to adjust the exercises and self-talk depending upon the situation and what quality I have chosen.

What about "graduating" from this self-improvement program? Will there come a time when I can finish this work and put all of these tools behind me? In my experiences, the answer is no. This work never stops as I am continually learning and adjusting to new issues in life. My need for new knowledge and skills is never ending. However, I find the work is not arduous; it has become a part of my daily routine. Furthermore, I can see real, concrete results. My payoff is improved health, which is like a dog getting a bone for doing a good job. In this case, the bone I receive is improved physical and mental health, and this keeps me going.

Chapter 11— Managing Immobilizing Guilt

Anger, fear, and guilt are all responses to a threat. When the threat seems stronger than me or I perceive it as overwhelming and unfair, I sometimes resort to fear and anger or a mixture of both. I add in guilt when I somehow assume I am at fault for the situation or I should have been smart or strong enough to have prevented it or reversed it once it started.

This parallels the common statement that there are only three basic ways to cope with any threat: fight, flight, or freeze. An appropriate translation of these would be: fight equals an *angry* response; flight is a response of *fear*; and freezing in place is what happens when I paralyze myself with *guilt*.

The genesis and persistence of these three dark moods suggest how I can reverse or heal anger, fear, and guilt: by working at various ways to manage, reduce, or neutralize the threats (to any degree). *As long as I fully understand that I have psychological "weapons" to manage (not necessarily cure) the symptoms, then the actual threat diminishes. I am empowered by the awareness that I can influence these destructive emotional responses over time.*

Guilt is my experience of embarrassment, self-loathing, humiliation, and unworthiness because I have failed to live up to a certain criteria. In simple terms, I feel guilty because I failed to live up to some standards set by myself or possibly by another. How significantly I experience the pain of guilt depends upon how aggressively I decide to punish myself. I could enforce the violation in a thoughtful manner or be ruthless and unforgiving in my self-discipline.

There are two ideas I consider when working with guilt. The first point is to evaluate the standard I have set for myself and determine if it is reasonable or not. The second issue is managing the rigidity and intensity with which I discipline myself. For example, I could have violated one of my standards and not feel guilty at all, because I felt it unnecessary to enforce. On the other hand, I may hold this standard in high regard and choose to enforce it aggressively, which could result in excessive guilt, mental, emotional, and physical pain.

My approach to managing guilt begins with the same 7-step process that I use with anger and fear. This dialogue with myself is a starting point that brings a level of control to my overzealous immature desire to achieve unrealistic standards. I need to approach this childish part of myself and take over the responsibility of both evaluating my standards and disciplining myself should I fail to meet the standards.

I have learned that my immature guilt-ridden self does not do a good job at setting realistic and achievable goals and is overly aggressive in his discipline. Unfortunately, he believes unrealistic levels of achievement and living up to rigid standards is the basis for his self-worth. This results in tremendous emotional turmoil and irritation that dumps itself into my gut and feeds my internal inflammation—destructive to me as a Crohn's patient. *Another name for the source of my guilt is my inner critic.* My inner critic has become overactive, too intense, and even tyrannical. *His unreasonable standards and unreasonable methods are a major source of trouble, requiring my skillful and firm attention. He repeatedly sets me up to "fix the unfixable" and "cure the incurable"—a recipe for disaster!*

So how do I re-evaluate these internal standards I have set out for myself? I start by making sure I am in a calm state and have worked through the first three steps of the 7-step process. I cannot clearly evaluate a situation when I am feeling overwhelmed. When I am calm and centered, I start my internal dialogue of wisdom, love, and giving perspective while asking myself questions, looking to see what "rule" I violated and evaluating the self-punishment inflicted. For example, I can ask, "What is the standard I have failed to live up to?" or "Can I reasonably live up to this standard or ideal?" Finally, if I have not met my standards, I can ask myself, "Does the punishment fit the crime?" meaning, "Am I being reasonable with my self-discipline?"

Here is an example as it relates to Crohn's disease: I am at home and in pain with a Crohn's flare. My daughter asks for help with homework and I do my best to help her, but my flare makes it difficult. As I go to bed that night, I wrack myself with guilt that makes my flare even worse. I can evaluate this as follows: the rule I broke is, "I will help my child 100% of the time." Of course, this standard is absurd because nobody can be perfect all of the time. This smacks of extreme perfection and I need to eliminate this unreasonable standard. My next question is, "Are my heavy feelings of guilt for not helping my daughter a reasonable punishment?" The answer is no because I did my best and that is all that can be done. I would have preferred to be more helpful to my daughter but I was sick. From this analysis, I felt excessive guilt because I was not able to live up to an unreasonable standard. Thus, I need to create a more reasonable standard and eliminate my punishment.

Let me now give an example of a standard not set by myself: my boss gives me a goal that is impossible to achieve and I fail to meet it. I feel guilty about my failure. As I look over the situation, I realize the goal was not achievable and it is ridiculous to punish myself for something that is unachievable. I need to release my internal angst, perhaps approach my boss to discuss his unrealistic expectations, or consider other ways to manage this issue without guilt.

Some people might argue that guilt is necessary and a good dose of guilt, like a good dose of anger, is healthy. I have heard people say that guilt forces us to be more self-examined and keeps us on the "straight and narrow." Guilt means that we care about others; it forces us to strive for higher goals. I can understand these arguments and relate to them. Self-examination is a critical component of personal development and an excellent approach to self-improvement. *However, strong and constant guilt, just like strong and constant anger, is destructive as it aggravates my inflamed gut and does not guarantee that I will be a better person. Guilt is not required to be a good person of integrity.*

For example, I could continually be condescending to others, which would violate my standard about how to treat people, and then feel guilty about it. However, this does not guarantee that I will do anything to remedy my behavior. I could continue being a nasty and difficult person and then feel guilty while never doing anything to fix myself. Feeling guilty does not guarantee that I will take action and work to do better the next time. I have met many people who are always sorry for what they have done but never do anything to change their behavior or try to make amends. They believe that being sorry is good enough.

I have asked myself where these unrealistic expectations came from. A main reason for my guilt and perfectionist standards was to please others, including myself, and have others accept me. I can still faintly hear the distant adult voices of family and friends from the past that were never satisfied with my performance and felt nothing I did was ever quite good enough or done correctly. Every statement of praise they followed with a "but" that said I could have done more. My own attempts to take it up a notch in order to appease these voices were never successful. I was not quite good enough in the eyes of certain people, or at least this is what I perceived. I do not believe my friends and family intentionally tried to harm me but their input resulted in feelings and thoughts of unworthiness when processed by my young and undeveloped mind. I think others were trying to help me improve and inspire me to greater heights. However, I just heard their voices of criticism and not of acceptance.

Ideally, as I grew older, I could have reevaluated their standards or my interpretations of what they said but unfortunately, I did not. As decades passed, the voices created by various people faded away but I replaced their voices with my own powerful "inner critic." This voice is the "immature or childish self" within me and I never learned to challenge what it said or turn it off. As an adult, I am now mature enough to work with my guilt-ridden self, come up with reasonable standards, and eliminate the unattainable ones that create mental pain and suffering.

I have also learned to stop spending time thinking about or contemplating other people who might have been overly punitive to me in the distant past. This is not the time to relive the past and dig up unhealthy memories. Reliving old or even more recent hurts makes me feel worse and does not solve my problems of today. *I remind myself again that my own voice of criticism is now creating the problem, not voices of others from my past.* I have to be cautious about my lifetime attempt to please either current or older authority figures, some of whom have disappeared from my life decades ago. At some point, I must step out of their shadows (and their rules, ideas, standards, expectations) and be my own person. This means that, while I still might prefer their approval, I no longer need it.

This could create a new problem: as I change and become my own person, others in my life may not appreciate my sudden change to being more self-guided. They may be upset because I no longer live by their rules and thus am no longer under their control. However, any consternation I face is a small price to pay for being in charge of my life with my own set of rules and guidelines. This is the way I need to function in order to manage the bullying nature of Crohn's and my inner critic.

Another scenario I need to manage is violating my own reasonable standards. This means my standards are good and reasonable, but I violated them. Does this mean it is now okay to feel exceptionally guilty and really turn the screws on myself as part of my punishment? While I could decide to feel guilty and hammer myself, this is unhealthy, especially if it is excessive guilt. After all, guilt does not remedy the situation. So what do I do? My answer is to use the experience of my failure to learn and improve my skills. *When I have violated a reasonable standard, be it from me or others, I strive to improve myself, ask others to help me learn new skills, make amends if I have hurt another or done a poor job, and take responsibility for my actions.* By doing all of these things, I am in a better position to avoid future mistakes while being a person of integrity and good conscience.

Let me share two very simple examples to illustrate this point. Taking my medically necessary medication is a reasonable standard, but I have failed to do so from time to time. Alternatively, I have lost my self-control with a friend when they did not agree with me on an issue. Now, I could shriek at myself and feel bad about either of these situations, but a better approach is to accept responsibility for my errors and create a program to correct my actions. It is important to treat a lapse in good judgment as something to correct without hysteria, fussing, or more guilt. It is like falling off the proverbial horse, I just need to get back on and keep going. With any inappropriate emotional outbursts or other poor decisions on my part, I address the issue, make amends, and move on with my life versus letting the guilt and self-loathing eat away at me. I must renew my commitment to doing the right thing and creating better tools to prohibit these future mistakes.

Here's another example: I have been excessively irritable to my family because I had a lot of pain with Crohn's. I recognize my behavior was out of line. What should I do? I could create more shame and guilt for myself, but this just makes my gut worse and does not help anyone. Instead, I need to recognize I violated my reasonable standard that says, "I will be patient and kind with my family regardless of how

Crohn's disease is behaving." I ask myself what I can do to avoid this in the future. I can work on my own self-control, communicate better with my family, tell them how I am doing, and make amends by expressing my regret for my actions and taking responsibility. In the future, if I feel too exhausted or on edge to maintain my self-control, I can excuse myself from the situation before I unleash my irritation on those around me. *In all of the above examples where I have been at fault, I may still feel regret for my actions—but I do not need to escalate to excessive guilt whereby I feel like a worthless piece of trash for my behavior and my gut ends up in spasm and pain.*

By having my adult self take on the role of creating my own standards and finding better ways to self-discipline, I have freed up the childlike part of me to do things that are more appropriate. My adult self has learned to take responsibility for my mistakes in a mature manner, thereby helping quell my excessive guilt, inner critic, and the corresponding heat and fire that aggravates Crohn's disease within me.

Likewise, I can diminish my disease-related guilt by reminding myself that the ultimate "cause" of Crohn's is probably genetic, environmental, or resulting from an unknown chemical and genetic imbalance in my body. *While I do not cause Crohn's, I can aggravate it by my immature responses, my neglect, or my efforts to deny that I need to do anything about it other than suffer. When I correct these mistakes, I have no rational reason to feel guilty about my Crohn's any more than I should feel guilty about a rainy day.*

One last thought. When I think of the three emotional experiences that cause me the most guilt, anger, and fear, I remember a scene from the movie <u>The Wizard of Oz</u>. Dorothy, the Scarecrow, the Tin Man, and Toto are walking along the yellow brick road and find themselves in a dark part of the forest. Everything looks creepy; even the trees seem sinister. At some point, they start to speculate what might lurk in the forest around them. What might be out to get them? As they start to talk about various bad scenarios, they conjure up the most frightening things they can think of: lions and tigers and bears, OH MY! They repeat this phrase until they work themselves into a frenzy and at that moment, a lion jumps out and they scream. Yet a few moments later, as the lion is harassing Toto, Dorothy pops the lion on the nose and the lion starts to cry... turns out he is not the monster they thought he was.

This story serves to emphasize a point. *My own thinking causes my issues with anger, fear, and guilt. I created them and they hold no power over me unless I let them.* If I continue to see these emotions as terrible and difficult to manage, they remain significant in my daily experiences. As long as I see them as an obstacle, I cannot overcome them and see them as just a part of who I am, I remain in their clutches and subject to their whims. Yet if I can see them for what they are—my childish attempts to manage a complex life and my inability to come up with more mature options—I am able to pierce their power and am no longer under their heavy sway.

This also reminds me of the scene near the end of <u>The Wizard of Oz</u> when Dorothy throws water on the witch, who slowly melts. I consider the water symbolic of the purifying effect of ridding myself of excessive guilt, anger, and fear. With regular attempts at quelling these nasty emotions and the use of purifying and healthy thinking processes, I am able to melt them into a pile of harmless goo. This requires consistent and committed work on my part to communicate with my childish or undeveloped self. My work is not finished in a day, week, month, or year. It is a lifetime of work, just like my experience of Crohn's. If I am to make strides in healing my entire being, I must work at healing my emotional and mental self too. By doing so, I help my character to grow and mature while reducing the fire of inflammatory emotional responses that burn me internally.

Chapter 12 — Dealing with Distorted Beliefs

I previously wrote about how Crohn's disease would behave if it were a person. He would be a bully, harassing people and giving them grief. My childish self has reacted to this bully of Crohn's, and other difficult life circumstances, with anger, fear, and guilt. However, by using my adult mind versus my childish self to better handle my reactions of anger, fear or guilt, my health improves.

Having handed off the management of my emotional and mental health to my mature adult self, what else can I do to create health? How can I effectively keep my angst at bay by using my higher mental faculties? *My next step: examine my internal beliefs as they relate to Crohn's disease and life in general.* Over time, I have mentally constructed a variety of beliefs and rules to make sense of the world. These are my own personal laws that I live by, including my beliefs about the physical universe as well as my psychological beliefs. Some of my beliefs are reasonable and healthy, but others are toxic and lead me into more despair and irritation. *My beliefs are the tinted glasses that I use to view my life with Crohn's and I must evaluate and correct them as necessary. The wrong beliefs continually recreate my distress of anxiety, gloom, pessimism, anger, hopelessness, apathy, or guilt even in the absence of any new scenarios or physical symptoms.*

For example, as a youth I created my belief that a doctor's office visit was painful and though this experience had long passed, I retained a sense of fear when I went to the doctor years later. I also maintained the belief that my Crohn's disease was likely to become worse and out of control, even though this rarely happened. My beliefs actively participate in promoting or sustaining distress even when the scenario has passed. On the other hand, healthy beliefs—such as believing that I can manage a situation and others are helping me with my disease—will improve my well-being.

In this chapter, I will delve into a number of beliefs I have created that revolve around Crohn's disease. I have chosen beliefs that have contributed to my own mental and emotional inflammation and thus to my physical distress. I am not exactly sure where these beliefs came from, but I know that my doctor, health care provider, friend, or family member did not create them. No, I created these beliefs on my own. I assume that (like my negative emotional energies of anger, fear, and guilt) I created these beliefs by using undeveloped, "immature or childish elements" of my personality. My beliefs were probably well intentioned, to keep me safe and make sense of the world. However, they are not healthy and I need to either modify or eliminate them.

These unhealthy, immature beliefs result in and reinforce my automatic negative reactions to distress and symptoms. Because I am passive and give little thought to my responses to life events, these habits take over when I am on autopilot. As a child this is about all I could do, but as an adult, I need to: 1) assess what is happening, and 2) come up with a creative, mature response versus my negative automatic reactions. Until I realize that I do not have to be a passive bystander to my own illness or other life situations, nothing will change. But once I recognize where I can take charge of my responses to life, I can open the door to therapeutic changes.

Limiting thoughts and beliefs

1. I am a victim of this terrible ailment. It is not fair.

This belief was my attempt to blame someone or something else for Crohn's since I did not want to blame myself. This is a toxic belief for two reasons. It takes me "off the hook" for having to fix the problem because I did not create it. It also says I am not as blessed or fortunate as others are because life has dealt me a terrible physical illness. This fatalistic and nasty belief becomes stronger when I am in the midst of a flare while other people are enjoying themselves. While they are out having a nice dinner, I might be stuck in the bathroom or in bed. This belief fuels my anger, frustration, sadness, and victimization. I realize that its poisonous tendrils are something that I need to rethink, reprocess, and change.

Seeing Crohn's disease as my life's curse causes me to fixate on the ailment as an integral, defining part of myself. This is like viewing a rosebush and putting all my attention on the thorns versus the roses. A healthy attitude is to identify with my strengths and potentials, not weaknesses and problems. I want to center myself in my resources and good possibilities—not what drags me down.

The truth is that Crohn's disease represents a real but only a small part of my life. My life is full of family, friends, career, various creature comforts, a good working mind, and an otherwise healthy body. I need to remember good fortune is evident in many areas of my life and that everyone has challenges to deal with. It might be health, relationship problems, career, or money issues. Living on the planet Earth brings challenges and obstacles of one kind or another. It is not a matter of *if* I will have problems in life; it is only a matter of *when*, what form they will take and what I will do about it.

Thus, I have chosen—and it is a choice—to change the above belief about Crohn's. I am not a helpless victim; I am an empowered creator of my own life. While I might have Crohn's issues to deal with, other areas of my life are rich and rewarding. For those areas of my life that are challenging, this is a call for me to do something about them and use my mind and resources to manage problems to my best ability. My focus will be on making the most of my life in spite of living with a bully like Crohn's disease. *Thus, I choose to change my belief from "I am a victim of this terrible ailment and it is not fair" to "I have many great things working in my life. I can find new ways to manage Crohn's disease and have a productive and joyful existence."*

If I am going to make this belief come alive in my life, I must do the mental work to convince myself this is true. I must be firm that this new belief is accurate and the old statement of victimhood is not, for it only represents a narrow slice of my life. *As my old belief comes up, I need to catch it early and remind myself this is no longer the way I am going to think. I accomplish this shift by quietly reminding myself of the abundant evidence of good things, achievements, and positive experiences in my life.* I need to do this repeatedly and over time engrain these positive thoughts strongly in my mind. If I fail to do this, my belief will not change and the ugly head of victimhood will continue to harass me forever with its pessimism and gloom. To this day, when I am feeling sick or tired, my old immature thinking will sometimes speak up and argue with me that I am still a victim. However, if I have really done my homework, I can rebuff this old belief and reaffirm my new conviction that I no longer need to wear the irritating robe of helpless victimhood.

2. My doctors will take care of me and I can relax. I just need to let go and let God take care of things.

These two beliefs are actually connected and they both revolve around the idea of what my role is in handling Crohn's disease. Here are some questions to consider:

- Is it my job to be active in managing the physical, mental, and emotional aspects of Crohn's disease, or do I have a more passive role?

- Am I to take charge of the situation and use my mind and body to create better health, or am I to rely on someone else to do it for me?

- Is creating better health a cooperative venture, or as a patient do I have few responsibilities?

- Do I readily acknowledge that I have an issue to deal with, and is it my job to participate in gaining relief?

While it would be nice for someone to phone in a cure for me, I realize this is not how life works and I cannot afford such laziness. My old approach was passive: I just wished and hoped I would get better, versus taking action. I would go to my doctor and let him know what my issues were and I expected him to fix everything with little effort on my part. My old idea of faith was similar. I was giving my problems to God and saying, "Fix me!" which was my passive approach to healing.

So how did this belief work for me? It took me 38 years before my diagnosis and many more years of suffering before I was finally able to create an improvement in my health. This belief resulted in substandard medical and personal intervention and many years of unnecessary pain and disability. If I had pursued better health years ago by being more proactive, I could have avoided additional inflammation and damage to my intestines or at least taken advantage of the best technologies to handle it.

So what is the best way for me to work with doctors or use faith to heal? *My best approach is one of cooperation.* Through cooperation, I do all I can to manage myself. I eat well, take my medications, pursue all avenues of treatment, and comply with my doctor's orders. With faith, I labor hard to clean up my mental, emotional, and physical health and work to incorporate new qualities of Spirit. As I do my part, I then ask for help from Spirit or God in my time of need. This program of cooperation has worked well and I consider it a central reason for my improvements over the past few years.

Based upon these positive results, I have changed my belief. I replaced my old belief of *"My doctors will take care of me and I can relax; I just need to let go and let God take care of things."* My new belief is, *"I will do all that I can to heal my physical, mental, emotional, and spiritual self and then work with my health care team and higher power to heal all parts of me."*

3. Because I am ill, I have the right to get special attention and freedom from certain responsibilities.

This belief, like the previous one, does not readily create strong experiences of anger, guilt, or fear but it is still damaging to my health. This belief works in the following way:

- Crohn's disease is uncomfortable and creates some disability.

- People are sympathetic to my plight and want to be supportive.

- Sometimes I will use my morbidity and sickness to get special attention even when I am not overly distressed.

I think this is normal for most people and it is okay for others to pamper me from time to time. However, if I use my chronic ailment to get frequent special attention on a regular basis, I am manipulating others and not doing enough to help myself. Reaping the considerable potential of special benefits of being sick also diminishes my interest in pursuing health and healthy activities. *Everyone wants to avoid severe distress and disability, but there can be an unhealthy allurement to remain less than fully healed since full healing would involve taking on a full adult role with all its responsibilities—and that would not be as much fun.*

Some people might argue that being ill gives them the right to special attention and I would agree. This disease can be very wearing and exhausting. However, if this belief becomes a habit, it would be easy to "take advantage of others" as an excuse to do less, shirk my responsibilities, and not look for better ways to mend. I become a less ethical person and an unnecessary burden to others while running the risk of not taking a leadership role in my own health. I consider taking charge of my health to be a critical part of managing Crohn's disease

I have taken my old belief of *"Because I am ill I have the right to get special attention and freedom from certain responsibilities"* and replaced it with, *"Because I am ill, I sometimes need the special attention of others. However, I will do all I can to take care of myself and be an advocate for my own health."*

4. I feel dreadful today and it will only get worse.

This is the total product of my feelings of disappointment and pessimism. I should not let these inferior departments of my emotions have control of anything I am or do. This belief comes up when I am in the midst of a flare or a long period of misery, which could include times when my personal or professional life is also experiencing challenges. I might feel bad with pain, cramps, nausea, or fatigue. I can allow this dysfunctional belief of never-ending suffering to escalate to the point when I start to think this illness is going to continue forever. As my thoughts of pending doom further escalate, I can easily generate a massive amount of fear, anger, or frustration, which further perpetuates this catastrophic thinking.

I need to be especially diligent to keep this belief corralled. I must catch this thought as soon as I notice it pop into my mind, for its anxious nature breeds even more anxiety and misery. Assuming I have caught it early, I take a factual approach to diminish this distorted conviction. I can look at my physical history of being ill and ask myself: what is the normal length of my acute episodes, and do I survive in good shape? By reviewing my memories, I can show my mind how I have been in distress before and come through in good shape even if a surgery or hospitalization was required. I tell myself that while I feel bad today, have felt this way before, and will likely feel this way again, there will be brighter days ahead. The harassing nature of Crohn's is knocking on my door and while it might get bad or even worse, I am a survivor and will be just fine by using all my resources.

This internal compassionate conversation in my mind calms me down and throws cold water on this agitating belief of despair and my irritating reaction to it. I am certain this belief has a strong connection with my "childish or immature self". It was simply my presumption that my current misery is "natural" and expected, so the only thing I can do is endure it. I thought there was nothing for me to do but suffer in helplessness—I had no strength to fight, so I might as well give in. It was a classic example of "the boy who cried wolf" telling me that bad things are here and it will only get worse.

I have created a new more accurate belief to replace this old one and it goes like this. Instead of believing, *"I feel dreadful today and it will only get worse,"* I replace it with, *"I feel dreadful today, but with my skills and the help of others, I will get through this and be all right."*

5. *I am a Crohny and my Crohn's disease defines me.*

This is an odd belief and it snuck up on me over time, before I even realized it. This belief is as follows: some time ago, I learned I have Crohn's disease and that this lifetime chronic ailment requires attention and regular treatment. As I took all of this in, I started internalizing this information and it changed the way I defined myself. As an example, I used to see myself as Jim who does this type of work, has this family, likes these things, has these interests, enjoys this faith, and sometimes needs to take some time off for his health. *Crohn's behaved like a cancer as it started to squeeze out other experiences and opportunities. I could see myself walking up to a new person and, shaking their hand, say: "My name is Jim and I have Crohn's disease." My world had shrunk, and this reduced my zest for life and hope for the future.*

So how did I work on this belief, which was defining my life in terms of illness? I thought about my life and the role of Crohn's Disease. I started with my body and found my organs and systems were all functioning well except for a chronically inflamed small portion of my bowel. I then looked at other parts of my life including my ability to communicate, my interests in art and music, my home, my education and learning ability, my family, career and friendships. These areas of my life more completely defined me, even with my vicissitudes with Crohn's disease.

When the bully of Crohn's disease roars and makes himself known, the rest of me must accommodate him. This is like coming in from outdoors when there is a thunderstorm. The rain, thunder, and lightning might change my plans for the day but I can go indoors and find other things to occupy my attention. *There are many situations that I need to accommodate but they do not have to define me, consume all of my interests, or squash my opportunities.* Does that mean I can do everything I want even if I am struggling through a flare? The answer is I cannot. Crohn's disease can limit my life in certain ways, but I can also maintain a fruitful and productive life. I have Crohn's

Disease and must deal with it, but the disease does not define me. My life is more than trips to the doctor, pain, procedures, or surgeries and Crohn's need not be my main topic of conversation with friends and acquaintances.

I am more than Crohn's. In fact, I am more than my body, mind, emotions, or even spiritual self. I am a multidimensional being with many opportunities to explore and things to experience. Ultimately, how I live my life becomes a choice and my choice is to accommodate the bully of Crohn's and live a full life. Thus I have chosen to change my belief that *"I am a Crohny and my Crohn's disease defines me"* to *"I am a multidimensional being with many different parts. I can have exciting life experiences while still accommodating this ailment."*

6. *I give up.*

There have been times dealing with Crohn's when I was not improving. I was exhausted and thought to myself, "I give up." My desire was to roll over and let this ailment run me down and take whatever crumbs of comfort, joy, or happiness remained. This dismal belief is very irritating and comes when I am most vulnerable due to an outbreak of pain, nausea, or frustration.

To manage this, my approach is to reason with myself and look at the situation carefully. I remind myself that I have experienced tough times in my life, bounced along the bottom, been tackled by either Crohn's or something else, but each time I got back up and moved on. I recognize my thought of "I give up" is premature. I have not yet turned over every stone or explored all my options. There is more to do; I am simply exhausted and worn out for the moment. I need to take a brief break and let my mind and body rest, as the idea of doing more work on my health is too much for now. *Any significant and chronic distress can wear me down, and I have periods when I get tired of being sick and the limitations it entails. This is a combination of my impatience mixed with fatigue. When I am irritated by my lack of progress, I need to reassure myself that 1) I have already done many things (diet, pills, meditation, etc.) to contribute to my healing, and that 2) many healing changes are occurring deep within myself—not currently visible, but soon to manifest physically and emotionally. Therefore, I can relax a bit and face my future with sensible and confident expectations.*

My next step in dealing with this belief was acknowledging that I do not have to heal in one day. I can take this big project of healing myself and break it down into manageable, bite-sized pieces. My mind can now take a deep breath because it can work on my health at a reasonable pace.

My bite-sized approach to health issues is to review what I am doing. I can revisit my medical options and possibly make an appointment with my doctor. Maybe it is time to talk with him and let him know things are not working well and I need some new options. I can also look at my mental and emotional work and see if I am missing something. Are there some distorted thoughts and beliefs or emotional energies that are getting out of hand and need to be changed? Perhaps I have not done enough work to build health and develop new qualities of character. Maybe I have been remiss in my spiritual work and need to recommit myself to growth. As I work through this in my head, I acknowledge this is not a dead end and I can do more. Sometimes the new answer is better medicine, a minor procedure, a small change in diet, a mental or emotional adjustment, or a prayer. *Sometimes it is to do nothing and let a few days pass so I can rest; I am just exhausted and need to turn off my mind for a brief period.*

I am a very curious person and my curiosity has been helpful in handling Crohn's disease. An intense interest in finding healthier options has frequently brought me to something new. A simple example occurred at Costco. I was struggling with my weight and diet and while visiting the store, I came across a demo of a high-speed blender. As I viewed the blender demo, I saw no placards stating *High speed Crohn's Disease mixer!* or *Works well with Crohn's patients!* However, as I watched this blender gobble up all kinds of foods, I saw it giving my digestive system a leg up. It would do a lot of work that my digestive system could not and it would create an easy-to-digest blended food. My doctors had never discussed this option with me, nor had my friends, family, or fellow Crohn's patients. The simple act of blending food gave me years of stable weight and vitality.

(A side story here: a few years ago while staying at a hotel on the Upper East Side of Manhattan, I had prepared a good morning meal of blueberries, soy milk, dates, apricots, protein powder, and bananas and placed it all in my high-speed blender… but forgot to put the lid on. I spent the next two hours cleaning off purple stains from the ceiling of our hotel room. I cannot claim it all came off, so if you are ever visiting the Upper East Side of NYC and your room's ceiling has a faint purple tint, it is a brief reminder that a fellow Crohn's patient was there.)

To this day, my firm belief is there are always better options and things I can do to recover. I am not expecting a miraculous cure but I see any incremental improvement as a win. This habit of looking for better alternatives has served me well with Crohn's disease and in other parts of my life. Thus, I have changed my belief of *"I give up"* to *"While my current situation might be tough, I am confident that I can find new and enhanced options to help me improve and I can relax at the moment and rest."*

7. I am *"Perfect Health."*

This belief is a good example of an idea that did not help. I tried to develop this belief because others had suggested it, I found it easy, and it was based upon some New Age thinking I heard about years ago. The concept is as follows: I am more than my physical body, my mind and thoughts, or even my spiritual self. I am a multidimensional being that at its basis is a perfect expression of what its creator initially intended. I am thus compelled to see myself as this perfect intelligence and expression of it. By continuing to focus on this thought and continually reminding myself that I am "Perfect Health," I will experience Perfect Health in my life. This sounds like a mouthful, but the basic idea is that by telling myself, "I am Perfect Health," I will experience Perfect Health.

I worked with this idea several decades ago and put a lot of energy into it. After years of working with this idea, the inflammation in my gut remained and my sense of well-being did not improve. In fact, my well-being deteriorated and I felt frustrated because nothing improved. This belief might work for others but it did not work for me. The idea of seeing myself as Perfect Health was an alluring one because it was so simple. I just had to think this thought, fully believe it, speak it and act on it, and I would end up with this experience of Perfect Health. This is a very attractive approach and I wish it had worked.

As I think back, holding the thought in my mind that I am Perfect Health while my bowel was in extreme pain, I was bleeding internally, I was anemic and exhausted, and I was emotionally upset created a lot of internal turmoil. My mind was trying to accept a thought that had no basis in reality. As I worked on this belief, there were times I felt I was living in extreme denial, in a fantasyland, thinking crazy and delusional thoughts.

This belief is important to bring up because in my attempt to look for better options and ideas, I will come across some ideas that do not work. Some ideas might be very attractive like this one where all I have to do is believe to get better. I am open to trying any idea that is not harmful. This is part of my learning process and I have tried many things over the years that did not work. From smelly concoctions, to exotic oils, to fancy herbs, to special meditations and mantras like "I am Perfect Health," I have explored a variety of ideas in my search for better health. I expect that I will try and fail with other ideas in the future and some of my own current healing methods will go away because they do not work. This is my path of trial and error to building improved vigor.

I do have one strong warning: I have been guilty of waiting too long before moving on when things are not working and this has delayed my healing and, in some cases, made things worse. I have done this with beliefs, medications, exercises, meditations, and other healing modalities. I have learned that after a fair trial of a technique or drug, if it does not work, I need to discard it and look for other options.

However, I did not discard all of what I learned by thinking of myself as Perfect Health. I do have at my core a blueprint of perfection and a source of energy and intelligence that I can put to good use. I am a multidimensional being with great possibilities. However, I need to work with the idea of Perfect Health in a pragmatic way by doing my part and not being so passive. My passivity was the reason it did not work. I have found a way to make this concept more useful for me. I replaced my old belief of *"I am Perfect Health"* with *"I know that at my core I have a blueprint of perfection, energy, and intelligence. I will honor this and garner its support by being active in my healing process and doing all I can to build a life of better character and health."*

I carry not only the above beliefs but others as well that are associated with both Crohn's disease and my life in general. While some of these beliefs are destructive, I have others that are healthy and support my vision for better health. Such healthy beliefs include:

- I am confident in my ability to handle the difficulties of Crohn's disease.

- I approach each day as an opportunity to grow and be creative.

- My family, friends and clinicians support me.

These "healthy beliefs" are more than simple affirmations. They have power and authority as I readily accept and experience them as truths in my life.

I have other non-Crohn's related unhealthy or dysfunctional beliefs. These old beliefs include:

- I can never make a mistake.

- I must always fight when I do not get what I think I deserve.

- I must always get angry when I see bad things happen in the world.

- Life is hard and I have to learn to live with that.

- I must be fearful of things not going my way.

These unhealthy beliefs can send me down the rabbit hole of despair and result in inflammation in my mind and gut. I did not create these beliefs in response to Crohn's disease, but they generate the kind of irritation (emotional inflammation) that feeds Crohn's. This is another fruitful area for major healing because it implies that Crohn's disease exists within me—a complex, living, breathing personality—but is not the only issue in my life. *I can and do work on other beliefs not related to my Crohn's and this work significantly influences my well-being.*

In order to work with a distorted thought or belief, I must figure out what they are. What is the best way to identify a dysfunctional thought or belief? I find my powerful emotional responses are signals that I have "stubbed my toe" on a strong belief. My powerful beliefs generally elicit the most aggressive mental or emotional reaction. Thus, as I go through my day and notice myself particularly agitated by Crohn's disease or another life circumstance, I look for a strong belief or consternating thought associated with it. As I have discussed before, the thought or belief comes first, followed by my emotional or mental reaction to it. Thus, I need to look for the thought behind my emotional response.

It could be as simple as waking up in the morning after a

tough night of being in and out of bed with pain or other GI issues. If I simply recognize that it was a tough night, I will not make a bad thing worse. But, if my belief kicks in that says, "This is not fair" or "I am being picked on," I will respond with anger, frustration, or fear. I need to avoid this. Creating a habit of catching these aggravating beliefs and correcting them has done wonders to cool my irritated thinking.

Does this work give me immediate relief from my distress? It can but usually I have to work at it, although over time it is easier.

I created many of my strong dysfunctional beliefs decades ago. Still others were born out of mass consciousness as I bought into whatever the crowd believed, even if the crowd was wrong. Some of these types of mass consciousness beliefs include:

- All drugs are unnatural and bad.
- Doctors do not care.
- Insurance companies are trying to rip me off.
- Bad things happen in hospitals.

While there can be a thread of truth in all beliefs, these are unhealthy over-generalizations.

Working to change long-term beliefs is difficult. I have learned to live with them like a rock in my shoe. I have grown accustomed to the pain and never thought to do the work of taking off my shoe and dumping out the rock. My beliefs can be part of the defensive armor that I think is protecting me or they are a central part of my persona, even if they are outdated and destructive. As I work with beliefs, it is critical to gently approach this childish part of me and establish a dialogue in order to work through and eliminate them.

As an adult, I thought it would be easy to give up unhealthy ideas and beliefs. However, I can recall many a time when I believed my excessive anger and fear were justified even though they were tearing me up inside. My beliefs were also something I must defend at all costs, as they were part of my sense of self worth. I have learned to ask myself what is more important, my health or excessive negative emotions and destructive beliefs. By placing excessive anger or fear on one side of the balance scale and health on the other, I have chosen to exercise more self-control and change my caustic beliefs while no longer allowing fear, anger, or guilt to run wild in my life.

I have built up mountains of psychological dirt over the decades (dysfunctional beliefs, and thoughts) and it will take a long time for me to clean it away. It will require skills and knowledge to do so. I liken it to cleaning a stain out of fabric. With certain fabrics, I must carefully coax out and gently rub the stains so I do not destroy the fabric. Psychologically, I have deeply engrained stains of bad habits, ideas, and beliefs and removing them takes time to access them and then gently coax them out. If I tried to clean up the "stains" (my dysfunctional beliefs) in a short time, I would probably tear the "fabric" of my personality and cause internal chaos. I must be gentle but firm in my approach.

Crohn's can be draining and I am never certain when the bully of Crohn's will pay me a visit. Thus, I work on my distorted beliefs each day as they come up. It takes patience, kindness, and thoughtfulness to change my stubborn beliefs that are not responsive to simply telling them to go away. By doing so, I can make progress and thus create improved health in my multidimensional self.

Chapter 13 — Therapeutic Gratitude

Previously, I wrote about guilt, anger, and fear as examples of the negative ways I sometimes respond to the discomfort of Crohn's disease. These emotional energies aggravate a difficult situation and add more irritation and pain while hindering my ability to heal. Connecting and dialoguing with my departments of anger, fear, and guilt is critical to handling these unhealthy reactions. I communicate wisdom and perspective to my immature self with an attitude of kindness, patience, helpfulness, and sincere interest. This approach helps me better manage my negative emotional energies and reduce my destructive mental processes. I also identified a variety of beliefs that involve Crohn's Disease and discussed the importance of modifying and eliminating them.

My work thus far involves using my intellect and willpower to enforce change in my existing mental programs and responses to life. I worked to change my choice of beliefs and self-talk. This was helpful but it was not enough. I needed to bring in new powerful transformative energies that function as an antidote to my unhealthy beliefs and emotions while also creating new energies and opportunities for positive expression. As an antidote, they neutralize my poisonous beliefs and expressions of fear, anger, and guilt and create a more nurturing environment for healing my issues. As a transformative energy, they change the paradigm of my own consciousness.

The transformative agents I chose were gratitude, forgiveness, and joy. I will write about these three major virtues in this and the next two chapters: what they are, how I work with them, and the results.

The work with these transformative agents is profound; I use the analogy of a house in need of repairs and cleanup. The foundation of the house is strong, but over time, some hardware has worn out or become obsolete and there has been a lack of deep cleaning. The work of better management of my anger, fear, guilt, and physical body along with reworking my old destructive beliefs is the process of cleaning and performing these repairs on the house. When that work is completed, the house is more functional and comfortable. However, the use of transformative agents is like adding electricity and gas to the house: it changes the entire experience. I can now easily use the house in both the day and night. Appliances such as a TV, microwave, refrigerator, stereo, and water heater that were original equipment but non-functional, now come alive and make living in the home an entirely new experience. This is how significantly gratitude, forgiveness, and joy changed my experiences.

Gratitude creates a sense of feeling supported and nourished. When I am grateful, I am part of a greater whole and see life as contributing to my success, well-being, and health. I am aware of the generosity of life and I respond with gratitude.

This is a healing antidote for someone who is chronically ill and filled with uncertainty. Having gratitude as part of my mental makeup casts a healing light into all parts of my mind and emotions as it helps dispel the darkness of gloom, anger, fear, and guilt. *These dark moods and emotions cannot thrive in a world I perceive as full of abundance of good things.*

Gratitude magnetizes me to the blessings I experience. The more I express and observe gratitude and the blessings in my life, the more I experience them. Gratitude is not only observed or seen in human relationships but is evident in my body, mind, and the world I live in. I can be grateful to the people who help others and me by expressing kindness, patience, and thoughtfulness. I can be grateful for the generous gifts of much-needed rain, sunlight, beautiful scenery, music, and majestic mountains. I can also observe the generous nature of my physical body with its many well-functioning organs and systems. As I am grateful for all of these generous qualities around and in me, my life is easier, more abundant, and better nourished.

My plan to work with gratitude was to observe what gratitude is, how people and life express it, and then express it in my own life. I learned that gratitude is not an object I can touch, hold in my hands, or put in my pocket. Instead, gratitude is a type of energy. It is an attitude, a motive, and a dynamic way of viewing all of life. Gratitude has various qualities that I can experience and relate to such as nourishment, appreciation, beauty, compassion, connectedness, and generosity. Reading about gratitude and hearing others speak of it was a good start but I needed to make gratitude come alive in myself.

In order to build my gratitude muscles, I chose to observe and acknowledge the examples of gratitude in my life and then actively work with them. An example of this work was when I was at a local grocery store a few months ago. As I was checking out, the clerk greeted me warmly, asked me if I needed anything else, enthusiastically processed my items, proceeded to talk about how nice the day was and left me with a gracious smile. *As I strode into the parking lot, I realized this woman was demonstrating sincere generosity.* I put my groceries in the car, walked back into the store, and approached this clerk. I thanked her for her kind generosity of spirit and wished her a good day. While her kind and generous behavior was a pleasant part of my day, my acknowledgement and appreciation for her service triggered joy, peace, and generosity in me. *The most healing part of this incident for me was actually not the clerk's actions—it was my response to her actions by observing her generosity and then acknowledging it by talking with her.* This was not a passive causal exercise, but a conscious effort with intent and energy to acknowledge her expression of generosity.

I make it a priority to add gratitude to my work each day. I have a number of people who work with me in the office. Their contributions and efforts are a critical component of the success of the business. They all contribute in different ways and have various levels of skills and experience. Collectively, they are the company and they are responsible for its accomplishments. They add value not only with their business-related skills and with creativity, but also with their kindness, thoughtfulness, and interest in those they serve and work with. I attempt to observe their contributions and whenever possible give heartfelt thanks for what they do. I understand that my own success and the working environment of the company are fully dependent upon their efforts and my appreciation for their efforts is important to foster a culture of generosity and gratitude.

Another example of working with gratitude was after I had my last major Crohn's surgery. After I returned home, I realized I had received good care while in the hospital but one nurse in particular had given me exceptional care. She was always there to help with a smile and took extra time to make sure I was in great shape. It was not just her efficiency and nursing skills, it was her commitment to patient care and having my best interests in mind. I realized she was constantly expressing a generous heart in all of her actions. Thus, I wrote to her hospital several weeks latter and expressed my thanks. The following is part of that note:

In my opinion, Wendy demonstrates an outstanding commitment to patient care in addition to her highly efficient manner. The best way to describe it is by example. I am sure that most people have been in a room and someone walks in, their warm presence immediately filling the room. Whenever Wendy entered my room, I could feel her kindness, thoughtfulness, and interest in my welfare. She did not even have to speak: her intent was clear. This was not work or a job for her. She was there because she was committed to patient care and doing all she could to help others. I was not a burden but rather someone she wanted to assist, work with, and help heal. It made a big difference to me knowing that someone cared and was intently interested. Wendy was exceptional and an important part of my healing process during my recovery.

My experience of gratitude was more than a simple thank you. I recognized Wendy's generosity, expressed my gratitude, and then experienced its healing qualities in my own mind and heart.

As part of my continued work with gratitude, I spend a few minutes each day recalling examples of support in my life and acknowledging my successes for the day. I recognize completing a big project at work, taking note of people thanking each other in a store, noticing that I had less pain that day, seeing the roses bloom in my garden, or celebrating feeling well and not needing to see my doctor. Looking for generosity around me has become my daily habit and as I become more aware of its presence, I experience it in my life.

At first, it was difficult to see generosity as part of my daily experience. This was because my criteria for observing generosity or expressing gratitude had a very high threshold. In order to see myself as being supported or thinking I should be grateful, I needed to win the lottery, have my bowel inflammation go away permanently, see my boss praise me endlessly, get a new car, have someone buy me lunch, or receive a large order at work. Big things had to happen in my life or I was not going to be grateful. The more mundane parts of my life where I felt supported were too trite to express gratitude for, and I ignored or took them for granted. I could not imagine life supported me unless events were out of the ordinary, sudden, or dramatic. For example, I rarely thought about a sunny day, having things go smoothly at work, enjoying a few laughs with friends, or experiencing a good night's sleep. *I took all these things for granted; I thought they were "supposed to happen." However, as my work with gratitude continued, I found countless blessings in the everyday parts of my life.*

I have been blind to my good fortune because my mind resisted the idea of feeling grateful for the small gifts I receive in my life. To solve this problem, I have used the simple exercise of opening my eyes to the nourishing world I live in. I can see the world's generosity in the abundance of food at my table, a completed project at work, or kind words that come my way. This includes being grateful for having a kind and thoughtful wife, listening to a concert, petting a friendly dog or watching a good movie. As I live these experiences each day and acknowledge them, I feel the powerful energy of gratitude course through me. These small gifts became my daily healing salve, creating healing and joy while reducing my internal inflammation in both mind and body.

Over months and years of regular practice and attention, this work has become easier and my experiences grow more profound. Generosity and gratitude come alive in all parts of my life. *As I connect with this ever-present support and nourishment, my mental state shifts from, "Life is a struggle" to "I feel supported in all aspects of my life."* I have learned to observe the many people who live their lives with confidence, ease, joy, and peace; watching these examples of gratitude further magnetizes this energy to me.

This work has helped in my healing work with Crohn's disease. When I am in a negative mood, I feel a loss of control and a sense that life is difficult and challenging. My stomach churns and this creates even more physical and mental pain. *Seeing my world in a generous light and expressing gratitude produces a deeply nourishing energy that comforts me in my areas of need and counters my internal inflammation. It brings forth the healing energy of caring, appreciation, supportiveness, and thoughtfulness.*

When I first started with this work, it was forced and mechanical. Much of what I did was to offer a pleasant platitude or a simple thank you. Over time, it has blossomed into a continual awareness of the generous and giving nature of life.

I have engrained gratitude in my life as a constant belief rather than something I have to work to remember. In addition, these internal changes have helped take away some of my pessimism and sense of loneliness and isolation. As a result, I am more optimistic and connected to the natural flow of life. Gratitude has enabled me to be more grounded and stable in my mood and expectations.

As this work with gratitude continues, some of the results have been surprising. For instance, I sleep better and feel more confident. Little things do not bother me as much. All my experiences are richer and fuller. Gratitude is like adding a super-charger or high-octane fuel; it takes all of my uplifting experiences and intensifies them.

While learning to observe and recognize gratitude in my life, I have worked to express these experiences as part of my daily living in different ways. I acknowledge gratitude by writing about it and working to make it my regular attitude. I look for new ways to express it by seeing it in my work and I look for examples of gratitude in art, movies, and literature.

Building gratitude into my character requires my full commitment. A half-hearted effort is not enough. It is not enough to work with gratitude only when I am happy or when it is convenient. My commitment to this work must transcend my whims or my moods. Just as I take the time out to eat or sleep, so too I must take time out to work with gratitude. Only then will it grow. I find it similar to exercising in order to build up my physical body. I cannot build physical muscles without regular exercise; nor can I build gratitude without seeing generosity in my life. This requires a motivation born of a deep sense of appreciation and a reverence for the quality of gratitude. I had to see it as invaluable—a true healing force in the world and worthy of my daily attention. I had to acknowledge it and express it in my thoughts, speech, actions, and attitudes. I had to do this regardless of my state of physical or emotional health. Only then, did gratitude help me to reduce the fear, anger and guilt associated Crohn's disease.

This work did not generate immediate results. I did not wake up one day full of unending gratitude, seeing the full generosity of life. This was because my mind did not believe this work would be effective and transformative. I was skeptical because I had many years seeing life as a struggle and full of painful challenges, including Crohn's. In spite of my own doubts, I did the work anyway and was surprised at its power. *As my experiences of generosity and gratitude have become more pervasive, I am no longer hopeful this will work—I KNOW it does, based on my own experience.*

While I have learned of the world's generosity and giving nature, I am aware I still have difficult issues in my life. There is still some imperfection around me and I will need to manage those issues. I liken it to my rose garden. There are always some weeds in my garden or thorns on the bushes, but my primary attention is growing and feeding the roses and as I do, I enjoy the beauty and fragrance of their blossoms.

My work with gratitude remains in its early stages and I have more to do. However, it has reduced my levels of fear, anger, and guilt and has given richness to other areas of my life. It has significantly reduced my level of internal irritation that can aggravate my experiences of Crohn's disease. My sense of well-being and lightness has increased and the bully of Crohn's is *less powerful.*

Chapter 14 — Healing with Forgiveness

My early experiences with forgiveness were less than enthusiastic or sincere. I can remember times when a friend had ridiculed or taken something from me. A parent or authority figure would tell the person who offended me to apologize for what they had done. The offender would look me in the eye and say, "I am sorry." In my young mind, I was usually not convinced they were truly sorry; I presumed they were only sorry someone caught them! They were apologizing because a nearby authority figure was forcing the issue. As a child, when my friend said they were sorry, I did my ritualistic part and replied, "It's okay, I forgive you." The expectation was that this was the end of it and the slate was now clean; however, I rarely felt better after this exercise.

There were times when the roles were reversed and I was doing the apologizing and not enjoying it either, especially when I was innocent or felt humiliated and embarrassed by my mistakes. My lasting impression was forgiveness is a laudable ritual but I rarely saw or experienced healing from the process. My gut remained tense while the heat of my irritation, anger, or fear would continue to simmer within me.

Through most of my adult years, my thoughts about forgiveness followed the same pattern. There is the offending person standing mournfully in front of the victim. There is the asking for forgiveness and the victim magnanimously accepting the apology and releasing the offending person for their transgressions. However, it still seemed like the pain and irritation remained while there was no healing. The exercise of forgiveness resulted in little more than lip service to the concept.

Then there are the public displays on TV, in some TV courtroom, or in a newspaper when a lofty public individual is caught in deceit or corruption of some sort and they appeal to the masses for forgiveness. The offender professes to take full responsibility for their actions and there is the gnashing of teeth and wailing of emotions. While some of these displays are sincere and heartfelt, others seem questionable and manipulative. These episodes left me with a feeling of distaste and cynicism around the quality of forgiveness.

Some people claim that litigation is a suitable method that bypasses the need for forgiveness. We extract a pound of flesh in the hope that this will heal the wound and bring inner peace and the sense that all is right in the world. The winner of the litigation might leave with more dollars in their pocket, yet the pain and hurt remain—and might even become worse when the public display reopens wounds. *This is not healing when one's gut remains in knots or when anger, fear, or resentment continues to prevail.* All these examples weighed heavy on my mind when I thought about forgiveness and its potential to heal.

Forgiveness must be a great quality, I reasoned, because noted philosophers, public officials, and key religious figures have mentioned it as a quality "par excellence" for centuries. I wanted to understand why. I could not work with a quality I did not respect because it would not heal me. I needed to find a better way to view forgiveness and rehabilitate this quality in my mind.

My first step was to understand the difference between forgiving and forgetting. I can forgive, but I will not forget. Remembering an event is generally useful and an excellent tool for learning. My memories of previous events allow me to review the situations and find better ways to manage issues in the future. For example, I can remember the signs and symptoms of an impending flare of Crohn's disease and this allows me to respond appropriately to handle it. By contrast, *forgiveness is when I stop directing my anger or irritation towards others, and it continues in what I do to make amends, how I heal my wounds, and motivates me to find better methods of self-control. Forgiveness does not mean I have to befriend those who have violated me, but it does mean that I have chosen not to direct my own angry energies towards them and have made peace within myself.*

Forgiveness must include my sincere attempt to make amends for my offending actions. Making amends might be through physical, monetary, or verbal means. I must be honest with myself as I observe my mistakes and the mistakes of others and put it all in perspective. I take stock of my errors, acknowledge them, and put together an action plan to make sure they do not happen again. This is likely to include managing my own impatience, jealousy, anger, pettiness, unreasonable expectations, or frustrations. I commit to cleaning up my immature character flaws while creating better ones like joy, gratitude, patience, or faithfulness.

Having defined forgiveness, my next step was establishing the criteria of what was worthy of an act of forgiveness. I observed that my threshold for giving or asking for forgiveness was too varied and inconsistent. If I was the violated victim, my bar was low and the violation required restitution. My criteria also varied depending upon who had violated me. If it was a family member, they deserved some leniency; relations that are more distant, strangers, or big businesses were not likely to garner any mercy at all. However, if I had offended another, the bar for giving forgiveness was high because it was my offense. I rationalized that I was not that bad of a person and perhaps had just made an innocent mistake or error in judgment and nobody should be upset with that.

My inconsistent criteria demeaned my concept of forgiveness. I must have a single set of criteria for what constitutes unacceptable behavior. Why would the person at the store, on the freeway, at school or work not deserve the same respect and forgiveness as those closer to me? Should I not do everything to make amends and then stride to be a better person to all? *I find it intellectually dishonest to have an inconsistent standard when working with forgiveness.* While this is a tough concept to live up to, setting the same standards for everyone is required for me to work with forgiveness as a laudable quality. Otherwise, it is nothing but an empty platitude.

The next step in cultivating forgiveness was to review my expectations of the other party involved with the issue. The other party could be a person, a company, the government, or even my own inflamed bowel in Crohn's disease. My questions were:

- What is the role others play in the process of forgiveness?

- Will they readily forgive me for my transgressions and be lenient?

- When they are at fault, will they feel deeply sorry and want to apologize?

- Will they do all they can to make amends and work to develop better self-control?

My concept of forgiveness involved having the offending parties fully participate in the process. This was an unrealistic expectation. Instead, the offending party might tell me to get over it or just ignore me. If I offended another, the other party might not want to hear my interest in making amends and instead remain angry and irritated at my behavior or actions. I learned forgiveness is my work and I cannot demand others' participation or even predict if they will participate.

I also learned forgiving others has nothing to do with cancelling a call for justice or demanding that others take responsibility for their own actions. Forgiveness is not my judgment on the behavior or event; rather, it is my decision not to pursue anger, resentment, irritation or hate in response. Bringing others to justice is not always within my control and I usually do not have the skills or insights to do so.

In the past, I used to think that directing my anger and irritation towards others who violated me would make them feel regretful and punish them for their errors. I felt I deserved and earned the right to be angry. I thought I had to keep directing my anger towards the offenders; otherwise, I was in effect saying that what they did was acceptable. This idea is incorrect. I have recognized that being angry or irritated towards others does not hold them responsible for their actions.

Directing anger towards others is another seductive belief that boomerangs back to me, making me ill with my own anger, irritation, and resentment. My directed anger towards other people or situations is destructive to my own self-interests. When I rant and rave towards my violators, I churn up all sorts of malicious energies that further irritate my mind and body. I have learned that as much as I want to lash out in frustration and anger towards others, I only end up being the loser. As a Crohn's patient, this keeps my internal inflammation alive and damaging my body. My anger towards others does little to change others or my situation but it certainly fuels the fire in my belly and pain in my mind.

If others violate me or if I feel humiliated, embarrassed, and worthless from making mistakes, I am likely to respond with strong feelings of anger, fear, guilt, or other unhealthy emotions. Underneath all of these harsh emotions are my wounds that tell me others have violated me or I hurt others. This is when I use my 7-step program or Emergency Mental Toolkit (EMT) as discussed in previous chapters. I use these programs to process and help heal my wounds. This is an integral part of working with forgiveness. After I have done some work to peel back my anger and fear while healing my exposed wounds, I am then able to bring in my adult mind to complete the work of forgiveness.

Having now established what forgiveness is, eliminated some of my false assumptions, and assessed how I manage the related negative emotions, I was ready to work with forgiveness in specific situations and memories. My goal was to use forgiveness to reduce the level of internal irritation and inflammation that aggravates my Crohn's disease, and to improve my character and overall well-being. My work with forgiveness involved several different scenarios.

In my first scenario, I saw the need to forgive acts of nature or genetics, which in my case was Crohn's disease. I had long considered how unfair it is to be stuck with this nasty disease while others are not. I directed my anger toward the disease within me. The bullying behavior of Crohn's disease had stolen some of my peace of mind, created mental and emotional pain, and disturbed my relationships and work environment while creating uncertainty in my life. I felt victimized by my own body and my irritation soon led to more stomach pain and discomfort.

It became obvious that I need to forgive what I viewed as a betrayal by my body. I needed to cultivate a broader understanding about what is going on so I could let go of my angst and irritation and forgive my body. Here is a snapshot of the internal discussion that went on in my mind as I worked to heal this issue.

"While I recognize that my gut is not working well, there are many other parts of me that are doing great, like my kidneys, lungs, mind, legs, heart, etc. My body is sound and supporting me in many areas. The parts of my body that are healthy far outnumber the parts that are ill."

"Other people just like me have parts of their bodies that give them challenges. Almost everyone has at least one issue to deal with—be it mental or physical. Having a medical issue is normal for many people, including me. I am not being singled out or alone with this problem."

"I have the ability to manage my ailment through mental and physical tools. With these tools, I can live a reasonably productive life while feeling supported and cared for. I have a great team of physicians, family, and friends and an inner intelligence to help me."

"Getting angry and irritated is very destructive and further irritates my gut. This type of reaction to my illness is poisonous and makes things worse."

This is similar to how I managed my belief that I am a victim of Crohn's. This type of mental discussion helps me to move beyond my department of anger and irritation and begin to heal. It helps me to forgive my gut and forgive "mother nature" for allowing this bully of Crohn's disease to be a part of my life. This takes time but it works if practiced regularly with sincere kindness. I perform this mental work with the calmness and loving attention that I would give a child. The irritation emanating from my "department of anger and fear" is *childish* and requires a soft, nurturing approach to manage. I must use compassion to help heal this wound.

This work gave me an astonishing revelation. As I worked with my adult mind and dialogued with myself, I reduced my anger and fear and this exposed the underlying hurt and pain beneath my resentment of my physical problem. At some point in the distant past, I became aware that I had something wrong with my life. There was a deep psychological wound of sadness and remorse. I felt isolated and lost. My childish self took over my reaction to all of these problems and placed a band-aid of anger or fear over my wounds. *At first I assumed this was all due to my Crohn's disease, but as I began to perform the mental work of calming and giving loving attention, I found that there were deeper layers to my distress that spoke of my sense of abandonment. This is where true healing needed to occur.*

I also found it is important to forgive my inflamed bowels. I had to do this in the same manner as I would when caring for a sick child or adult. I needed to give them mental encouragement and emotional support along with good food and nutrition to nurse them along. There is nothing to forgive, for they did nothing wrong but unfortunately have taken ill. I must treat my ill intestines as I would any illness—with compassion, sensitivity, and nurturing.

I recognized that I would frequently be upset at my inflamed bowels. I yelled at them and told them how bad they were. This was hurtful to me. When I would rage at my gut, complaining about how bad it is, I immediately experienced a tightening in my belly and more pain and distress. This proved that my body "hears" me yelling at it! Thus, I recognized the need to supply encouragement and loving support instead.

The next scenario I worked on was my irritation when I am a victim of another person, group, or organization. For instance, I felt violated by a doctor who did not listen to me during my appointment. My situation occurred many years ago when I visited my doctor and presented my issues of pain, discomfort, and anxiety. I remember he took a cursory look and then rather flippantly told me there was nothing wrong. (He was wrong, of course.) As I left, I felt wounded, angry, and violated but took no action either to find another physician or manage my anger. Instead, I just stuffed it inside, considered it my fate, and carried around this bitterness within me.

I have now learned better ways to handle these types of issues. Using my new tools, I would first assess if I presented my case fairly and accurately to my doctor. Had I responsibly done my own homework before the visit? Did I feel that my doctor had really done his best? It might be there was little that he could do for my issues and my expectations were unreasonable. The other possibility was my doctor was rude, ignored details, or did not take the time to listen. However, my doctor is human too and perhaps had a bad day—just as I do from time to time. Or, I might have been particularly vulnerable on that day and my need for TLC was unrealistic; if so, I would need to "shrug it off" and move on without expressing anger or irritation. Ultimately, if this doctor frequently behaves this way and does not give me the attention that is reasonable, I have the choice to either confront him or get another doctor. In this case, I eventually took action and changed doctors.

If this situation occurred today and I felt some small wound from my interaction with my doctor, I could also use the 7-step program described earlier to manage the issue if needed. I would release my need for retribution or retaliation and focus on healing my own wounds so I do not carry around another bag of irritation. By doing so, I release myself from the toxicity of these emotions. *I would not wait in earnest for the other party who inflicted damage on me to come forth with an apology commensurate with the violation.* I can gain perspective by considering that others are not intent on making me miserable, and it is not a personal attack.

Most of my internalized anger and fear are born out of many small, poorly managed issues. Over time, these issues and baggage have accumulated and filled my mind and body with excessive anger and grief that burns me inside. The solution is to frequently recognize my angst, think it through, and take whatever mental healing steps are necessary to stop the accumulation of any "new mental baggage."

One other concept I have learned is the need to "give up" my right to apologies or compensation for long-past injuries, wounds, and losses. I have made too much of how my old wounds and injuries began. My life should not be about how bad things began, but how I finish—that is, what and who I have become in spite of violations is what is important. This is more than just letting go. It is seeing the value of no longer demanding reparations, holding onto my anger, or creating misery within myself. Each time I dip into old hurtful memories from years or decades ago where I have chosen not to forgive, I stir up fresh experiences of anger, irritation, fear, or self-pity. It never stops. *Reliving old memories and ruminating about past negative issues comes back to hurt me. It is the gift that keeps on giving.* If needed, I can use the 7-step program with my old memories to reduce the anger or fear, expose the hurt, and heal. There are enough challenges today without digging up old issues that cause me pain.

I have met some people who are challenging to be around and work with. They carry a constant chip on their shoulder and are obnoxious, derogatory, and insulting. I recognize this type of behavior is unacceptable and try to shield others and myself from its impact. However, I must share the planet with difficult people and they are part of my humanity. These people have their own issues and part of my life experience is to learn to manage myself as I deal with difficult people. I know there is generally little I can do to change them, for their behavior is their choice. However, I do have the option to respond in a more controlled way. I realize these are people like me who are trying their best but are frequently unaware or insensitive to the damage they cause. They are temporarily blind and cannot see the results of their actions. Through my work with forgiveness, I have learned to be more understanding of these personalities, as I see part of them in me.

In the next scenario, I am not the victim of bad people or bad situations—I am the victimizer. I was in the hospital fresh post-surgery and my wife was helping me clean up. For no good reason, I snapped at her for being too slow and forcing me to sit upright for too long and aggravate my pain. I lost my self-control and spewed out anger towards her while increasing the fire of my own irritation, pain, and spasm. My wife had done nothing wrong and was trying to be gentle and helpful, yet I insulted her. I was way out of line. At that moment, I did little to rectify the situation although I mumbled an apology at some point. I understand she may not respond or accept my apology. (However, she did.) I have now learned to handle this type of situation differently by immediately offering an apology, making amends, and committing myself to fix the issue. I have learned better ways to exercise self-control so these negative emotional outbursts do not exacerbate my Crohn's disease while alienating those around me.

Working to correct any areas where I have made mistakes or wronged others eventually leads to self-forgiveness. Some people think we should not forgive ourselves for our own mistakes. The idea is that we are flawed human beings and thus will always make blunders. Therefore, we need to remind ourselves of how imperfect we are and the mistakes we have made. Forgiving one's self might lead to becoming a narcissistic person who has no concern for others and is not able to see and learn from mistakes. I believe this criticism of self-forgiveness is nonsense.-

I have learned that self-forgiveness is essential for healing. My life has been full of mistakes and I will make more. Remembering my mistakes is invaluable but I can learn to avoid them in the future by developing various new skills. However, remembering these mistakes should have no connection to berating and whipping myself without end. My condemnation will not make a better person. I become a better person by recognizing my errors, making amends, finding better ways to handle the situation differently in the future, and building new skills. This is lot more than simply saying I am sorry and asking for forgiveness.

Constant criticism beyond remembering a simple mistake will cause massive mental irritation and self-loathing. It will leave me stuck in an endless cycle of unworthiness that will make me less able to help myself or anyone else. Self-forgiveness allows me to heal myself, learn my lessons, and still feel worthy. I no longer see mistakes as a failed part of my character because they now serve to motivate me to become a better person.

By acknowledging my own transgressions and making amends, I have become more understanding of others. I realize that others are just like me and have their own issues and faults to deal with. Just as others do, I have bad days and do stupid things. Knowing I am a work-in-progress helps me to become more empathetic and understanding of others. I realize we are all here to learn and we do this primarily through our mistakes and managing life's various challenges. The mistakes I make are a call to make amends and improve myself. *As I note my own mistakes and ask for the forgiveness of others, I become more understanding of my own lack of self-control and errors. This makes it easier for me to forgive others for their mistakes as I see parts of my own immature and out-of-control self in them.* I see us as equals of the same humanity and birthright.

Working with forgiveness extends beyond the many examples of Crohn's disease. I use it with the following real issues:

- my loss of self-control in personal and professional settings

- the humiliation and embarrassment of failing to live up to reasonable goals set by myself and others

- my forgetfulness

- my inability to effectively keep up with those brighter, more attractive or creative than I am

- my experiences of others bullying, taking advantage of, insulting, or neglecting me

All of the above issues can result in strong condemnation of others and myself; relieving myself of this internal cancer of distress requires all my tools of forgiveness.

I have worked with forgiveness with the difficult issues of my personal life, rather than large global disasters. I have not worked on the huge unforgiveable catastrophes in life. I consider myself to be in forgiveness "elementary school" and the unforgiveable catastrophes are "college level" stuff. What goes on around me in daily life creates plenty of opportunities to restrain my temptation to "feed" my irritation, fear, or guilt with poor self-control. However, I am certain that the principles I use to manage my anger or fear can also be used to manage big global events. I can separate the events, as terrible as they might be, from my reaction to them and know I can do nothing to change anything in my past, the past of others or the world. *Being permanently angry and upset might help some people validate that they have a legitimate gripe for their apparent victimization, but this is a massive price to pay in terms of internal mental irritation, bitterness, and self-pity while there is no healing.* I cannot see long-term negative emotional reactions to such events as productive and healthy to an individual or society; the anger and bitterness just prolongs the pain. In addition, for me, the irritation of Crohn's disease is exhausting enough without intentionally adding more into the mix.

My work with forgiveness has surprised me with additional improvements in my character. It has not shut off all my emotional responses or made me into an unfeeling robot. It does put me in better control and helps with my responses. While some anger, irritation, fear, and guilt continue, I am better able to manage these responses. Working on forgiveness has made me more understanding and flexible as I recognize how people learn from their mistakes and are generally doing their best to improve their own humanity. I have become more sensitive to others who have their own issues and are trying to work through them. I can see that others are often not intentionally trying to be harmful but instead have simply failed to recognize the negative impact of their actions.

The deeper value of working with forgiveness is that it connects me with my own humanity and with the humanity of others. Forgiveness makes me aware that I am one of many striving for self-improvement, better character, and amends for past mistakes. I am working along with others to find new ways to accentuate healthy qualities such as peace, joy, gratitude, humility, and kindness and applying them to reduce anger, fear, doubt, worry, and guilt.

It brings to my mind the painting "The Creation of Adam" by Michelangelo. I see this painting as an archetypal image of a higher force reaching out to help a lower force and the lower force also extending his hand to reach upward to get help from the higher force. I realize each individual with their own lower qualities of anger, fear, doubt, and self-pity are reaching upward to touch more noble qualities of goodness, kindness, self-control, love, joy, and peace. These qualities seem to come from a higher intelligence contained within us, accessible to us as part of our birthright. We can learn to express them. As people collectively embrace and work with these higher qualities, they are able to reach back down and help those on the same path to overcome their less-than-noble qualities. This is a fundamental principle of the compassion of forgiveness: we all need help and make mistakes while we collectively strive for higher principles and qualities. As we develop these noble qualities, we can in turn help to lift others alongside us.

Chapter 15 — Creating Joy

Joy has always given me pleasant thoughts, but for years I was not sure exactly what it was or how to work with it as a healing agent. Like gratitude and forgiveness, it was something that could not be touched and held but I could observe its effects and experience it. I use a similar process working with joy as I do with gratitude. *I need to expend energy and effort to build up my "joy muscle" by understanding, observing, and expressing it.*

I recognized that joy is not the same thing as happiness. Happiness is a response to an occurrence or event. For example, my response to winning the lottery, having a new baby, buying a new car, or developing a new relationship could be happiness. Something has happened in my life and I responded to that with happiness. My experience with happiness could also be the result of small events like getting a phone call from a friend, tasting a new food, or getting a compliment from my boss. All of these experiences are pleasant; happiness means I feel good inside. It is like mental thumbs-up. Happiness is something I look forward to in response to positive events in my life.

Yet as enjoyable as my reactions are to good events, I am stuck having to deal with difficult events and issues too. Examples of these could be getting a speeding ticket, failing a test in school, missing a promotion at work, chipping a tooth, having an argument with a friend, making mistakes, or having a Crohn's disease flare. I do not enjoy these events and would likely respond to them with anger, fear, sadness, or disappointment.

I am thus stuck with swinging between good events in my life, which make me happy, and undesirable occurrences, which make me upset. This pendulum swings me back and forth depending upon the blowing winds of life. This happens with Crohn's disease, too—one day I feel great with little pain, and the next day I am in bed. I can also make a bad day worse by responding to a bad event or situation with even more anger and irritation.

Thus, joy is not the same thing as happiness and is a unique energy unto itself. Joy has some similarities with happiness: it can elicit pleasant or uplifting sensations and it tends to make me smile and feel peaceful, contented, and supported. However, joy is not my reaction to an event, but instead is a permanent quality that is independent of my outer circumstances. It is an energy that is part of my character. It is with me when I wake up each morning and go to bed each night. Joy is there in good times, bad times, sickness, and health. *The strength and power of joy is that it is there to see me through the tough times and weather the various challenges and storms of life. Joy is my port of calm and a necessary ingredient in my management of Crohn's disease.*

I observe and experience joy in a variety of ways. With joy, I feel nurtured and cared for. Joy is playfully optimistic, putting a sparkle into everything I think about and observe. It creates confidence that life is benevolent and can be trusted. Joy colors all parts of my life regardless of the situation I am in, for it is a celebration of life itself. If I am going through a tough time, joy makes the angst less pronounced. If I am having a blah day, joy makes the ordinary routines more lively, interesting, and fun.

Joy becomes a very powerful ally as I work through the difficulties of Crohn's disease. It raises the valleys of my ailment and gives me hope and optimism for the future. It significantly reduces my psychological pain and thus reduces my physical pain. My feelings of struggle and pessimism are dispelled by the underlying optimism and celebratory energy of joy.

Having understood what joy is, my next objective was to observe it. In order to do this, I had to learn to put less attention on what is wrong in my life and the world. My constant habit of seeing the dark side of things was like wearing dark and fogged sunglasses. The only thing I could see with these glasses were grey shadows. Seeing the bright side of life is even harder when I am upset or ill; people seem more difficult, life is more restrictive, and activities are more arduous. In contrast, on days when I feel great, life seems supportive, magnanimous, friendly, and cheerful. Because of this, my observations of joy can vary depending upon how I am feeling. In order to overcome this, I need to use my objective mind to scout out observations of joy and not my emotions or pessimistic mind, which can negatively color my thoughts on the day.

Joy is not a tangible item that I can pick it up and study directly. However, I can look for and observe its expressions in the world: combinations of optimism, nurture, playfulness, and celebration. The *following are some examples of observed joy.*

- I marvel at the joy from one of my neighborhood dogs. Every day is a good day for Kippy as he runs about sniffing and exploring the world. He welcomes the chance to visit and always greets me with affection.

- My wife has spent the last 37+ years greeting me each morning with a kind, "Good morning." Her amazing optimism and enthusiasm for each day is an inspiring example of joy.

- I can hear some people at work on the phone conversing with laughter and pleasure. They are chuckling and animated and this joyful energy lights up the whole office.

- I have several friends who generate great joy as they work with others and are helpful. They express joy as part of their service to others and their commitment to a noble purpose.

- As I approached my last major surgery, I noticed that my affect remained upbeat and calm even with a pending surgery. This surprised me but I came to understand this was active joy in my life. I would catch myself humming, whistling, or smiling for no reason other than being joyful.

- I can recall another example of joy when I was at a music event and saw an individual slowly walking towards her seat. She was bent over from the effects of arthritis, yet she continued to shuffle along with a gentle smile and a glow in her face. There was a joyful appearance of radiating health even in the midst of a crippling disease. Her joy was independent of her experience of arthritis.

Having worked at observing many daily examples of joy, my next task was to express it. Observing joy requires a focusing of my attention and curiosity, but to express it requires the use of my will. By expressing joy, I can turn it from an abstract thought into an active energy in my mind and thoughts.

I make joy active by working with its higher qualities in my actions, speech, attitude, and thoughts. I can write, talk, think, or paint about it. I can think about the qualities that joy represents and then try to work them into whatever I am doing. I can express joy by being more playful, enthusiastic, confident, optimistic, and benevolent. I can do this on vacation, at home or while taking a walk. I can do this even when I might not feel well or have had a difficult day. I can express joyful confidence that I will manage my disease well by being kind and thoughtful to those people who help me at the endoscopy suite, in the hospital, or at work. Joy is more than a simple mood or an emotion—I experience and work with it under all conditions. It is something I create by acknowledging that life holds countless great opportunities.

Another way I build and experience more joy in my life is through meaningful activities of service. By seeking to be helpful to others in a genuine and sincere way, I experience joy. I do this at work, with my family, friends, or any acquaintance as I look for something they might need and then try to help.

I also build joy in my life by speculating and anticipating the great opportunities available in my life. I can ponder on questions or statements such as:

- I am looking forward to tomorrow and what it brings.

- I am excited to see this project come to completion and observe the results.

- I am starting a new job and am enthused.

- I am interested in writing a new book and am thrilled to start the task.

In each case, I am not 100% sure of the exact outcome from the situation. These are all future events and I am speculating that the outcome will be favorable. In the past, I have struggled to be optimistic about the future. Even though my life has been successful, I have minimized it with my constant pessimism and outlook that events will turn out badly. This way of thinking has reduced my experience of joy because I have not emphasized the possibility of a positive outcome. *However, with my positive speculations of the future, I invoke more joy in my life. This is not the same thing as positive thinking. I build this form of speculation around my confidence that life supports and nurtures me versus just hopeful. I am speculating with a sense of calm certainty versus simple hope.*

Another tool I use to build joy is celebration. This area of my life has been woefully deficient. While I have accomplished much through getting a college education, having a good career, and doing my best in all my activities, I have not celebrated these accomplishments. I did not attend any of my college graduations and in general have ignored or given little credit to my life achievements. After I completed each task successfully, I immediately launched onto the next project with nary an acknowledgement. Life has become one task after another and while they have been marked with success, I have not celebrated. I liken this to making an outstanding meal and then not eating it, buying a new home and not living there, or buying a new car or TV and not using them. Even as I have won psychological battles like overcoming fear, anger, or guilt, I have failed to stop and celebrate these achievements. This lack of commemoration of current and past accomplishments has created an underlying sense that life is hard and full of drudgery and struggle.

My motivation behind not celebrating was that I thought it was a frivolous waste of time. This idea is wrong and contributes to my sense that life is difficult and not rewarding. I have learned to take time to celebrate my achievements and the achievements of others. My form of celebration has significant benefits that transcend simply having a good time and partying. Having a good time and partying are fun, but joyful celebration is more than that. True joyful celebration gives credit to the beneficent nature of life and verifies that more of the same is likely in the future. By celebrating, I am saying that life is rich and full of opportunity and this will continue. Celebration affirms that the nature of life is to grow and expand.

Celebration is an acknowledgement of achieving a level of mastery over a challenging situation or being a witness to creativity, beauty, or achievement. Celebration recognizes life's abundance, prosperity, and health and calls forth a joyful experience in response. True celebration pays homage to the world we live in and connects me to deep joy.

Finally, I have found it important to take time to notice and appreciate the good things that happen to me. Even small things like a beautiful sunset or a soft rain help me recognize that there is beauty and abundance in the world for others and me. By recognizing this, I can shut down my hyper-alertness of what is wrong or missing from the past and present. Appreciating life means I stop taking for granted what is good around me. This helps to remove my bias for disappointment and my bias against whatever is satisfactory. I spend a brief period at the end of each day reflecting upon:

- at least one instance when I experienced joy by observing the world around me

- at least one instance where I created joy by being helpful

Equally important is my investment in observing the joy I see experienced by others. They are my fellow humanity and we are intimately connected. I want to see the presence of joy and support in their lives, take notice, and celebrate with them. This initially was difficult to do. In some strange way, I felt that if others were receiving good support in their lives, this meant there was less for me. My mindset used to be that there is only a limited amount of joy and abundance in the world and if others are taking their fair share, then I have less. This "poverty" thinking was destructive to my own welfare and it bled negativity through all areas of my life. Furthermore, it contributed to my thoughts that said, "I will always be more sickly and diseased than others" or "Others will have more of everything than I will." I have been surprised and shocked to realize that by celebrating the joy and gifts that other people receive, I experience more of the same. This unexpected result has been a blessing and it speaks to the truth about joy and life's benevolence. There are no limitations to the amount of joy and goodwill in the world. We just need to connect with this goodness as it is expressed in others and us.

Working with joy, like working with forgiveness and gratitude, is not a weekend or special holiday event. In order to be developed, joy needs to be a part of daily living. It has to become a priority in my life and not just a simple exercise. My approach to working with these qualities has always started as a mechanical process but it steadily becomes more natural and a powerful heartfelt desire. In a strange way it is self-perpetuating because the more I work with them, the more interest and desire I have to further visualize and express them throughout my day.

In addition, as time passes these qualities are transformative; they become the glasses through which I view the world. I replace my glasses of darkness and murkiness with lenses of color and brightness. Life becomes lighter and easier, as if a burden has been lifted off my shoulders. It is a remarkable experience. Moreover, as I work with joy, forgiveness, and gratitude, my gloom and pessimism associated with Crohn's disease diminishes.

Finally, I often remind myself that the qualities of gratitude, forgiveness, and joy have always been present in my life even if I did not recognize them. They are in the earthly soil of my worldly existence and a normal part of the home I live in. They are the precious stones of my human heritage, my birthright, and are available to everyone. I need to mine them and bring them forth into the light of my mind. I can then do the additional work of polishing them—expressing their qualities—so they fully reflect healing energies into my life and the lives of others.

Chapter 16 — Spiritual Help

I have written extensively about how I work with physical, emotional, and mental components of my multidimensional self to improve my health by developing various tools and making changes in my mental software. The final component I chose to work with was my spiritual self. How do I define "spiritual self" and how do I work with it to help manage Crohn's Disease?

I will not be writing about religions, churches, religious texts or the clergy. I have a tremendous respect for people who have an established traditional faith and church. However, I cannot speak in these terms as I have minimal personal history with traditional faiths and church. I created my own program to connect with my spiritual self.

While I have not been involved with religious traditions, I always had a powerful sense that there is a benevolent and intelligent force orchestrating my life and environment. This is what I call my "spiritual self." I have distinct early childhood memories that there was more to life than I could observe. As I grew older, I could only rectify the complexity of the universe with the presence of an underlying active intelligence. It made no sense to me that the universe, with all of its diversity and intelligent design, could exist without some sort of higher force. I felt a strong need to tap into this intelligence and work with it to improve my own health and character.

I saw this underlying force behind my physical form as the true healer in my life. While there is a lot of science behind the mechanism of healing, the science does not explain why healing occurs or how it is created. I consider this underlying intelligence to be the master orchestrator of it all. This intelligence heals damaged bowels after surgery and heals my distressed mind with qualities of joy, forgiveness, and gratitude. This force has healed me in the past and will continue to heal me now and in the future.

After recognizing this intelligence in the world around me, I connected with it within myself. This is a very personal and intimate experience. I experience its healing powers and nourishment. While this intelligent force may be active in fields of grain, oceans, or distant lands, it is also active within me, creating qualities of joy and gratitude while facilitating the workings of my body.

This intelligence helps me to heal as I do my mental "housekeeping" and work with its qualities of forgiveness, gratitude, and joy. This intelligence further works with me as I express wisdom, patience, optimism, or peace. As I work with these qualities, I am tapping into this "spiritual help" and using it to heal my environment and myself. I have found many ways to connect with my spiritual self, which I will explain in this chapter.

I work with continuous prayer on a permanent basis. This connects me with this benevolent intelligence. This form of prayer is my personal commitment to do my best each day and ask for continual guidance. I focus on living with integrity, peace, joy, humility, wisdom, kindness, self-control, and love, and as I do so, I express gratitude to this intelligence for its help.

I also work with a more focused, abbreviated form of prayer. While my prayer could be lengthy and drawn out, I find that a short heartfelt prayer works well when I am working on specific issues. I expect this generous intelligence readily translates what I am trying to say without me having to go into a lot of detail. My responsibility is to do all I can with my mind, emotions and physical tools to help with my health and other challenges. Having done this, I ask for assistance and anticipate a response. I acknowledge that this healing force is the true source of healing in my life and then express gratitude for this gift of answered prayer.

This prayer works for me. I get real answers that translate into results. My answered prayers have not always lifted my burden or cured me in the way I expected. However, I always receive the strength to carry on for the moment and a better long-term solution. There were times I did not notice an immediate response but realized later that the answers were already in hand. There were other times when the answers to my prayers were hard to deal with and I wanted the easy answers. I have learned that the easiest answers are nice but sometimes my medicine requires significant effort or sacrifice on my part. For example, I delayed a needed surgery for years because I hoped for an easier option but in hindsight, the surgery was the perfect solution to my prayers for a very diseased and non-functional piece of bowel. In another situation, I wanted a simple resolution to a burdensome relationship but I had to first work on my own communication skills and self-control before it was resolved.

While I have many examples of answered prayer, the following is a remarkable, detailed story that involves Crohn's disease. A number of years ago, I was in significant distress related to Crohn's. Decades and decades of this ailment had worn me down. While I had tried many creative options, I was chronically ill and could find no new options to pursue. At this point, I put forth a rather urgent prayer that I needed help, as I was literally starving and filled with hopelessness. As I ran this prayer though my mind over a few days, I caught an internet announcement about an upcoming educational program for Crohn's patients at a local university. I had not attended one of these events before and did not see the benefit, but this time I got a mental nudge that said to go. I did not have any real expectations of what I would get out of it but I went anyway.

At the meeting, I heard some good talks but did not see anything novel or unique that would be helpful. I visited the booth exhibits and found nothing new. After lunch, I saw a face from afar that I recognized: one of the national leaders in Crohn's research as well as a practicing gastroenterologist. He has published more papers on Crohn's therapy than anyone else I had read. I approached him and introduced myself. After a few moments of discussion, I shared my case with him and he remarked that it was very complex, unusual, and challenging. He then looked me in the eye and said, "I can help you." I will always remember that moment. It had been a long time since I had heard those words. My doctors frequently told me to "hang in there," as they saw little else they could do. I was amazed at his quiet confidence. I thanked him for his comments but told him that his practice was two-thousand miles away and I could not get there. He explained that he had just changed locations and was now within a couple of hours from my home. He handed me his business card and told me to call his assistant on Monday and make an appointment.

One week later, this physician thoroughly examined me in his office. This was the most detailed exam I had ever experienced. He told me my therapy was inadequate and made some adjustments. Over the next year, we worked together to maximize my therapy and as my health improved, my optimism did as well. I consider my chance meeting with this doctor to be an answer to my prayer.

This is not the end of the story. A year later, while my overall health had improved and I had gained weight, I ended up back in the hospital with an obstruction that affected my liver and pancreas. As I lay in the hospital, I put forth the same prayer I had used the year before: that I was doing all I could but still needed help with this issue. Soon after, my new doctor told me that we had done all that we could do medically and the only way to improve was to have a complicated surgery. Because my last surgical result was not ideal, I was rather hesitant about moving forward. I pondered on this and remained uncertain how to proceed. I needed more assurances or further validation to take this big step with another surgery.

Then it dawned on me that I had already received my answer but had not responded to it. A month earlier, my beautiful wife Mary Lou was traveling by plane from New York back to California. As the plane was getting ready to land, she struck up a conversation with the couple sitting next to her, whose names she learned were Stu and Beth. Their conversation continued as they got off the plane and walked to the baggage claim area, where Stu told my wife that he had Crohn's disease. This resulted in a lively conversation of about fifteen minutes and then a hurried exchange of phone numbers before they zoomed off to rent a car. When I picked up Mary Lou from the airport, she told me of her pleasant but brief visit with this couple. She said we should look them up sometime when we are in New York.

Later that evening, Mary Lou commented that maybe we should get together with this couple while they were vacationing in a nearby city. I questioned her about having a dinner with people she had only met for thirty minutes on an airplane. Neither of us had ever done this before but for whatever reason, I felt compelled to say yes. We would get out and meet some new friends and I could visit with a fellow Crohn's patient. My wife called Stu and Beth and asked if we could get together the next evening. They heartily accepted our invitation and we drove to meet them and had a lovely meal and a grand visit. We talked late into the night and created some great memories.

However, the following is what stuck out from this meeting and I recalled it vividly as I pondered my need for surgery. As we ate and visited, Stu spoke to me about his extensive experiences with Crohn's disease. I found his information interesting and could relate to it. Then partway through the meal, he looked me in the eye and told me I needed to have a surgery right away with an exceptional surgeon. He said if I did, I would feel so much better. This became Stu's mantra to me for the evening: "Have the surgery and have it now with an excellent surgeon and you will feel better."

His message rang clearly in my head. Stu was the mouthpiece of this intelligent force via a chance meeting with my wife. The obvious message was, "Have the surgery." My prayer was answered in the form of a good new friend who cared about my welfare.

This still is not the end of the story. I now had the ideal gastroenterologist and a clear message to have surgery, but I still needed to find the exceptional surgeon. I was uncertain whom to choose but fortunately, when I requested the help of my gastroenterologist he was able to supply me with the name of a surgeon. This surgeon was not someone I had heard of but he had spent years specializing in Crohn's surgery at a major medical center and working with another leading gastroenterologist in IBD. This surgeon had also recently located to my area. My gastroenterologist said he would set up my meeting with this surgeon and I met him at a special time outside of the normal clinic hours. He took time away from a convention to meet me and we were the only two people in the clinic that day. After reviewing my case, he informed me that he could help although it would be a complex procedure. He shared with me how he would perform the surgery and felt confident that his many years of experience working with complex cases would pay off.

There is another twist to the story. Several days prior to my surgery, I had a vivid dream. In this dream, I saw my surgery performed in a very creative way. I saw my symbolic surgery in the dream as a choreographed ballet with everyone working together in concert and moving gracefully about. Several days later as I lay on the operating table, my surgeon told me that over the weekend he had thought a lot about my case and had changed his mind about what to do. He came up with a novel approach that he had not considered before and was going to perform the surgery that way. He was excited about his new ideas and ready to put them into practice. As I was about to be put under, the dream of several nights before popped into my mind and I realized this was the new choreographed event that was about to start. The surgery lasted over five hours but the results were outstanding. This surgery resulted in the best improvement in my physical health in thirty years.

I cannot prove an intelligent influence in this story. However, I find this series of events to be remarkable. There were many things that had to come together to make this work. Just by chance, I had seen the advertized meeting and decided to attend. By chance, this nationally known gastroenterologist was there who had recently relocated to my area. In addition, he asked me to drive down immediately to see him. Later as I struggled to decide whether to have a surgery, by chance my wife had sat next to a Crohn's patient named Stu on an airplane flight from New York City. We got together with these "strangers" for dinner when he told me repeatedly to have the surgery with a great surgeon. In addition, by chance, my gastroenterologist knew of a great surgeon who was new to me. He had recently moved to the area and he could take on my case. Finally, my surgeon changed his surgical protocol a few days prior to my surgery and created a new procedure that seemed to correlate with my creative dream imagery. Yes, you could call all of these events random chance—but I choose to see them as an active, personal intelligence working in my life.

Another short story of answered prayer was in New York City. I briefly wrote about this before. I made the mistake of eating some pistachio nuts and quickly became obstructed and very ill. As I collapsed on the sidewalk in the rain, I offered up an "abbreviated prayer" that I needed help. I was uncertain what I should do or where to go. My close-knit medical team was 3000 miles away and it was a weekend night. As I lay there in the rain, it came to me to have my wife call my gastroenterologist in California to see what to do and where we should go. We left a message on his call service but did not hold out much hope he would be on call as he was a part of a large group practice. Surprisingly, we got a rapid call back and it was my gastroenterologist. He just happened to be working that night doing procedures at the hospital. He asked what was going on and assessed the situation. He said I needed to go immediately to a specific hospital by ambulance that could handle my case. He stayed with us on the phone until I was in the ambulance. After I arrived in the ER, he called back and spoke with the attending physicians. He gave them the details of my case, the nature and severity of my illness, the types of testing that could be done and the interventions to consider. The ER doctors worked with me extensively through the night and were able to stabilize my condition.

Some of my stories of answered prayer seem mundane and do not involve Crohn's disease but are equally valid. I attended my sister's 1500-student nighttime high school graduation and while sitting in the grass in fold-up chairs, I lost a contact lens. I was unable to see it in the dark and as I left, I counted the row I was in and hoped to return the next morning to retrieve it. Upon my return at 8 a.m., all of the chairs were gone and what remained was a grass-covered football practice field. I spoke my brief prayer of help and proceeded to walk out into the field. Immediately, I bent down and picked up my dirt and grass covered lens. I was amazed but thankful that my simple and sincere prayer for help had worked.

Finally, I have one story that involves my college education process. A large university in the Midwest accepted me to their graduate school program in Biochemistry with a full scholarship. After several months, I realized the program was not for me. The focus of the research and academic interests were not consistent with my own. I felt dismayed and miserable by my poor decision and could not see any viable options of what to do. However, upon reflection, I thought to call someone I had worked with as an undergraduate student and he recommended that I drive about 300 miles to another large institution and look into their program. He gave me the name of a faculty member to meet. I followed his advice, quit my current school program, packed everything into my car, and made the drive. I "dropped in" on Monday morning, looked up this faculty member at the new university, and told him who had sent me. I expressed an interest to attend this school's graduate program and he told me I would have to apply to the school and then interview with some of the faculty. He was kind enough to let me do this immediately and I spent the next few days interviewing. As each day ended, I picked up some fast food and then returned to my car in the parking lot and went to sleep.

By Wednesday morning, the faculty member informed me they had accepted me into the graduate program and I was thrilled. However, I had no money for tuition, room and board. When I asked if there were any scholarships available, he said no. However, he did say several of the faculty members had funds to pay graduate students who worked in their labs. I spent the next few days interviewing with these faculty members and by Friday, they informed me that one of the faculty members had accepted me and would cover all of my college expenses, room, and board. They asked me to return in a few months to start the program at the beginning of the new quarter.

This story may not sound like much, but from my side it is quite remarkable. The opportunity to be accepted and given full funding to attend a major graduate program and have this all occur in one week while I slept in my car is noteworthy. The end of the story is I did well in the program and a year later this is where my wife and I began our lives together. This was answered prayer.

I think these examples of answered prayer are astonishing. *However, the answers to my small daily prayers are more common and equally enriching.* Life blesses my family, home life, friends, and me with a rich history of support. I can recount many days when unexpected good news and good results have appeared. Just today, I got an unexpected call from a client wanting to expand his business and use our services. Yesterday, I had an urgent health issue unrelated to Crohn's that needed attention and was able to see a specialist within three hours due to an unexpected cancellation at his office. Several weeks ago, another couple I know were having a particularly tough time. As I went over to see them that night, I picked up a small book that spoke of everyday people overcoming various challenges in life. I had not read the book but as I gave it to them, I chose to read them several vignettes from the book. Much to my surprise, the first vignette spoke of reconnecting with one's mother and the other story spoke of a challenging time in a particular war. It turns out the situations readily matched experiences each of my friends had in their own lives. We all felt as if we were reading about them in this book. The coincidences in these stories are, I believe, a message that an active wise intelligence is at work in the world.

I cannot offer up concrete evidence and prove the presence of an active intelligence behind these events but I can see the correlation between my request for help and the answers. There are many times when random events occur that I cannot logically account for and they all seem to be in response to my continuous and brief prayers of asking for help and expressing gratitude, forgiveness, and joy. *My answered prayer could be as simple as some kind words of encouragement when I feel down, help with a relationship, a new idea, a solution to a problem, or relief from an acute episode of Crohn's disease. This is what I need to live a fuller life.*

I find self-control, skillful effort, and self-sacrifice helps me to connect to this intelligence. I use all of these qualities to reduce my anger, fear, and guilt; develop qualities such as forgiveness, gratitude, and joy; and create better, healthier beliefs.

I have other tools that help guide my spiritual self. The first tool is my strong desire to work with it. Connecting with higher intelligence requires an intense interest on my part. Just thinking about it casually from time to time does not work. This does not mean that I must set aside a big chunk of time each day for prayer— instead, I live a life of continual prayer. Through continual prayer, each moment becomes an acknowledgement that I am supported and cared for by a personal intelligence and I do all I can to connect with it and live a life of self-control. I expect this benevolent intelligence will answer my sincere needs.

I expect support from higher intelligence but I know I must do my part. I do not expect my answered prayer will mow the lawn, do the laundry, handle a work assignment, deal with a head cold, or manage my own immaturity or departments of guilt or anger. However, it will heal and help me to make wise choices. For bigger challenges, I can pray for specific needs with the full knowledge that the best answers will become available to me. My prayer is more than just wishing and hoping.

Another tool I have found useful is my intense interest in developing my own character. The harder I work to clean up my own act and do my best, the more I feel supported by this intelligence. Higher intelligence responds better when I am calm, centered, and not full of anger, fear, or guilt. As I work to calm these negative emotions and incorporate new healing ones, I improve my connection with higher intelligence. I have learned that my emotions are magnetic and tend to attract more of the same. If I fill myself with anger or fear, my experience of these emotions increases, dampening my ability to work with higher intelligence. However, I experience more support and a deeper connection when I work with gratitude, joy, forgiveness, or patience.

I find that as I work to help others, I receive more support in return. I do not have any systematic instructions of how to do this. Helping others can be as simple as volunteering or helping my family and friends. It could include charitable acts throughout the day while at the grocery store, at work, while walking through town, or visiting with friends. Charitable acts are not always outward but can also be heartfelt, silent expressions of interest in others. My thoughts and attitudes are projections of my mind and, like radio waves, they have an impact even if they are not readily seen. As I ask for the best for others, I am invoking the help of this intelligence and it helps me too.

It is not only service to others that connects me to higher intelligence but also my service to principles. These principles could be integrity, honesty, kindness, patience, perseverance, forgiveness, joy, or gratitude. They could also be my commitment to truth, knowledge, goodwill, educating others, finishing a noble project, helping people at work or listening carefully to my children. All of these are universal principles and actions that have a significant healing power in the world and as I participate, I experience their healing energies too. As I commit myself to working with all of these principles and ideas, I find myself part of a larger entity and feel supported.

I connect to higher intelligence as I offer blessings of support to others and myself. This is especially true if I offer support to those people I find challenging to deal with. The same is true as I offer support and love to my diseased bowel or forgive myself for making a mistake. Offering blessings of support is easy when I feel good and work with close friends. Offering love and support to the difficulties in my life is challenging, but the results are powerful. I think this is because I am invoking forgiveness and as I do, the energy of forgiveness has an exceptional power to heal all relationships and issues. I have learned that as others heal, I heal as well.

I am not perfect and frequently create problems for myself through my own foibles and mistakes. The nastiness of fear, guilt, anger, and my immature nature raise their ugly heads from time to time. However, each day brings a new opportunity for service and expressing noble qualities, committing to higher principles, building my character, and helping to make a difference. I have found nothing more healing than this endeavor and I attribute this healing to the underlying support of a benevolent intelligence.

I can use the same analogy of a house I used previously to describe the impact of spiritual help in my "home" or life. I wrote about how cleaning up excessive anger, fear and guilt along with repairing negative beliefs is like repairing and cleaning a home and making it more comfortable to live in. Adding in forgiveness, joy, and gratitude is adding electricity and gas to the home, transforming it into a very dynamic place with many new options. Working with spiritual help is like adding in WIFI, connecting me to a network of wisdom and love. The WIFI is significant because it works no matter what room I work in. I could be working in the "rooms" of my career, health, family, or personal development. The WIFI of spiritual help works wherever I am and connects me to this vast personal and nurturing intelligence.

There are many other ways to work and connect with higher intelligence of Spirit than those listed here. I am not an expert on this subject but these are some of the methods I find useful. I continue to look for better ones each day. Working with this personal higher intelligence is a key component of my own healing process: indeed, it is the true healer in my life. I use my healing methods with confidence and expect results. I hope that the reader will explore his or her own methods to connect with this power and use it.

Chapter 17 — The Search for New and Better Answers

Crohn's disease is difficult to manage and requires creativity, constant surveillance, and courage. In this book, I have indicated what has worked for me, pointed out my mistakes, and discussed what I have created and learned. I have explained better ways to communicate and take charge of my own treatment by addressing this illness using my physical, mental, emotional, and spiritual self in a comprehensive approach.

There is no cure. Crohn's disease has a high rate of morbidity and the need for surgery is common during one's lifetime. Crohn's disease is like the weather; it can change day-to-day or even hour-to-hour. I need to be attentive and involved versus just hoping for the best. I must live with its bullying nature that is a part of me and find ways to accommodate and manage it.

I have learned that to work effectively with Crohn's disease I must continue to look for new and better answers. I need to ask questions like:

- What can I do today to improve my health?

- What is working and what is not"?

- What do I need to change today or stop doing?

- What other resources can I apply to make this situation better?

- Is there something I am missing or have ignored?

- How can I get through this difficult day?

I ask these sincere questions to myself and to the intelligence within me and then look for helpful answers. At first, this whole process was awkward but with practice, it has become a productive habit. I must be cautious of dismissing difficult answers such as I need to have a surgery, a procedure, or work to manage my out-of-control anger or fear. I would rather have easy answers such as I need to take a pill or get some sleep.

Does this mean that my whole day revolves around Crohn's disease and asking questions and looking for solutions? It does if I am having a particularly bad day, but more likely, I am simply checking in with my body and myself. It is like looking to make sure dinner is cooking well. It is not necessary to camp out by the stove, but you need to check often enough to make sure it does not burn.

Based upon the answers to my questions, I make small adjustments each day. I might feel compelled to eat less today or to call it an early night. I might skip on dinner and have some tea instead as my belly is a bit bloated. I could recognize I am obsessing with thoughts of anger or fear and I need to work on that. Sometimes I might feel some pain and reach for the Tylenol early so it does not get out of control. In addition, I now know the big warning signs of a serious flare and take action as necessary. The answers come throughout the day as I ask for them. I am ready to listen and respond, as they are my street signs along the road giving me options as to how to proceed.

While this type of questioning is productive, other types are not. Asking questions that focus on my frustrations and remorse are not useful. For example, the following questions are not helpful:

- Why did this have to happen to me?
- Why am I the only family member with Crohn's disease?
- Why does it have to hurt so much?
- Why do I feel embarrassed and humiliated by this ailment?
- When am I going to feel better?

These questions may give me intellectually interesting insights but I cannot use the answers to heal myself. These questions tend to send me into the misery pit of self-pity and depression. Asking why I have Crohn's disease and why I have to suffer is not helpful as it just further aggravates my mind and disease.

My regular practice of looking for better answers has become a favorite tool I use for personal growth. Intense curiosity is a wellspring of new ideas and solutions to many issues. I use these inquiries to search for better answers in business, relationships and with family, in addition to managing Crohn's disease.

As I review my many experiences with Crohn's disease, I note how I have responded with anger and fear versus understanding and support. This has greatly contributed to my distress. I learned this is a choice and what choice I make affects my health in a dramatic way. As I go down the path of more anger, fear, and guilt, I experience more of the same and my emotional and mental health declines. There is no law that says I need to respond this way. While responding with negative emotions to a bad experience might seem appropriate, it is a disaster. Self-control is a key virtue in dealing with Crohn's disease. It becomes easier as I clean up my old negative responses to Crohn's and incorporate new virtues such as gratitude, joy, forgiveness, and patience.

I have given considerable thought to my experiences with Crohn's, what they mean, and how they have influenced my life. I have experienced many challenges along the way and have grown through the process. It has driven me to develop better life skills, priorities, and self-control. Through my work on managing the bully of Crohn's, I have noticed improvements in my mood, courage, resilience, sense of purpose, and ability to put my attention on what is important. In short, I have become more comfortable with myself. Managing the bully of Crohn's has enhanced my emotional, mental, and spiritual muscles, and it has given me more patience, understanding, and confidence.

The nasty influence of Crohn's disease has forced me to transform myself to survive, but this transformation has yielded significant benefits. While it was possible to become defeated and pessimistic through all of this, living with a bully like Crohn's disease has been an exceptional learning experience on how to manage difficulty. It has made me conscious of what a bully is and how this type of behavior by others or me is counter to healthy human relationships. I have learned about my own inner critic and how its bullying nature contributes to my experience of worthlessness and a roaring internal inflammation in my gut. In spite of many surgeries, hospitalizations, and medical procedures, I am healthier overall—physically, mentally *and* emotionally—than I was decades ago. I have learned how to remain optimistic and enthusiastic about life and its possibilities.

While I have no other physical ailments beside Crohn's disease, I would expect this multidimensional program of health improvement to help other chronic ailments such as arthritis, chronic pain, or heart disease. Working to reduce negative reactions to challenging ailments and building new healthy qualities should improve the health of anyone—including those who are physically healthy, for there is more to health than a healthy body.

I have not cured myself of Crohn's disease and its bullying nature comes to visit occasionally or takes on some new form. Over the time I have written this book, I have experienced a brief flare that required a short dose of prednisone, some pain with adhesions, had an MRI, CT scan, colonoscopy and endoscopy, and passed a kidney stone. (Kidney stone formation is more prevalent in Crohn's patients than the normal population.) I have also made some minor adjustments to my diet, mental and emotional work, and schedule as needed. However, in spite of these issues, I remain focused on my health plan. The bully of Crohn's, while unwelcome, has not overwhelmed my sense of support, well-being, and mental health.

As with any plan, I must execute it to experience any chance of results. I will continue to use the program I have outlined in this book and look for better ways to manage each day with new ideas and processes. My hope is that modern science can find a cure for this ailment and permanently put to rest the bully that is Crohn's disease. In the meantime, I can live a meaningful life as I use better tools to quell the occasional outbursts and tantrums I face from Crohn's.

It is my hope that others like me will work to create better tools and processes to strengthen themselves and hold the bully of Crohn's at bay, while transforming their own lives with better self-control and many new qualities of character that will nourish them each day.

ABOUT THE AUTHOR

James Patterson is a California native and received a Masters of Science degree in Biochemistry from Michigan State University. He spent 14 years working for a number of clinical diagnostic medical companies in research and development and sales. James has spent the last 22+ years as a medical recruiter working with medical businesses on a national level to identify and hire professionals in roles that include research and development, sales and marketing, regulatory affairs, operations, manufacturing, and senior management. Life has gifted James with two beautiful daughters, an amazing wife of 37+ years, many encouraging and outstanding friends, exceptional work colleagues, and good fortune in many areas of his life.

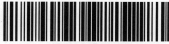

Made in the USA
San Bernardino, CA
11 May 2014